CLINICAL CT:
TECHNIQUES AND PRACTICE

THE L'R'

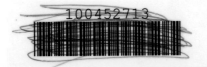

i

CLINICAL CT
TECHNIQUES AND PRACTICE

Edited by

Suzanne Henwood

MSc HDCR PGCE

Department of Radiography
City University, London

GMM

© 1999

GREENWICH MEDICAL MEDIA LTD
219 The Linen Hall
162-168 Regent Street
London
W1R 5TB

ISBN 1900 151 561

First Published 1999

British Library Cataloguing in Publication Data
A catalogue record for this book is available from the British Library.

Distributed worldwide by
Oxford University Press

Typeset by Saxon Graphics Ltd, Derby
Printed in Great Britain by
Alden Press, Oxford

CONTENTS

CHAPTER 4

The Thorax 47

Shelagh Smith

CHAPTER 5

Contrast Enhancement in CT 69

Peter Dawson

CHAPTER 6

The Abdomen 79

Sheila Rankin

CHAPTER 7

CONTRIBUTORS

Peter Dawson
BSc PhD MInstP
FRCP FRCR
Professor of Medical Imaging
Department of Imaging
Hammersmith Hospital
London

Sheila Rankin
MBBS DCH FRCR
Consultant Radiologist
Department of Radiology
Guy's & St Thomas' Hospital Trust
London

Shelagh Smith
BSc(Hons) PGCert DCR(R)
CTC
CT Superintendent
The Harley Street Clinic
London

Leigh Donnison
DCR DMU
Formerly ImPACT, now BMI
The Manor Hospital
Bedfordshire

Emma Spouse
DCR MSc
Superintendent Radiographer
MRI Unit
Torbay Hospital
Torquay

H. Szutowicz
HDCR SRR
Superintendent
Neuroradiographer
Addenbrooke's Hospital
Cambridge

Suzanne Henwood
MSc HDCR PGCE
Lecturer
Dept of Radiography
City University
London

PREFACE

This book is aimed mainly at radiographers with a working knowledge of computed tomography (CT), and its purpose is to increase their knowledge base to enable them to confidently play a proactive role in enhancing image production and writing new protocols, while constantly working to reduce radiation dose.

As CT hardware and software continues to evolve, its place within the imaging department remains secure. The speed and versatility of spiral CT has assured its role in radiology for the foreseeable future, despite the impact of magnetic resonance imaging (MRI) in certain areas, for example, bony spinal tumours.

For radiographers to remain skilled practitioners, they need to maintain their knowledge of anatomy and physiology and to continually update their knowledge of pathology, as well as being aware of equipment capabilities and protocol specifications. From 1997 this has been a requirement under the College of Radiographers Continiung Professional Development Policy [1] and will become a legal requirement with the revision of the PSM Act in 1998 [2].

With this wealth of knowledge, radiographers should play a full role in advising clinicians as to the most appropriate imaging available in order to gain a full diagnosis, while optimising imaging procedures in order to enhance the service given to the patient, including the reduction of radiation doses to a minimum. In the current cost-centred environment of the NHS, it is vitally important that imaging modalities are used to maximum effectiveness, and in order to do that skilled, professional radiographers are required to provide the specialist services of CT.

This book provides the information required for radiographers to adapt imaging protocols in CT, using commonly presented pathologies to show how scan quality can be optimised. A basic working knowledge of CT equipment and of the history of the evolution of CT equipment is assumed. The material concentrates on third- and fourth-generation scanners and on spiral technology, as most departments now have access to spiral scanning and most companies are developing the technique above and beyond other third- and fourth-generation operation mechanisms.

The book is aimed at helping student radiographers, especially those studying at postgraduate level, radiographers working in CT and radiologists who wish to enhance their knowledge of the practical, technical skills that can be used to optimise patient diagnosis in CT.

Each chapter looks at basic patient preparation and, although this is not explicitly stated, it is expected that professional radiographers working in CT would have excellent communication skills, especially given the physical distances between the radiographer and patient during practical CT procedures. Radiographers should optimise the use of intercommunication systems and make full explanations prior to leaving the patient alone in the room. It is also assumed that full explanations about patient preparation and aftercare are given. This book takes the radiographer to a higher level of knowledge and understanding without, it is hoped, patronising them in their current positions.

The use of contrast media is discussed in depth in Chapter 2. In addition, where appropriate, contrast is discussed within the topic areas throughout the other chapters. It is more important than ever that radiographers should understand contrast issues, as many are performing intravenous injections. It is essential that the questions concerning when contrast should be injected, at what rate, and in what quantity, should be understood and again, contrast administration should be tailored for each individual, to optimise image quality and patient safety. Radiographers should know how to calculate the quantity of iodine given in any one injection by using the simple formula;

$$\frac{\text{Strength of contrast} \times \text{volume injected}}{1000}$$

Other issues which are included in the text and need to be considered by the radiographer, are patient oriented problems. Patient positioning can be problematic, for instance if you are using CT to plan for radiotherapy of the pelvis (See Chapter 6. The selection of equipment will have to include consideration of aperture size, to allow the patient to keep their arms at their sides, and a flat table top will need to be employed to mimic treatment positioning, otherwise a repeat scan will be required by the radiotherapists. In contrast, routine chest imaging requires patients to raise their arms above their heads, a position which can be difficult to maintain; what can the radiographer do to optimise both imaging position and patient comfort ?

Patient preparation, especially for abdominal scanning can be vitally important and the radiographer should know how to adjust preparation for each individual considering size, metabolic rate and pathology. Abdominal preparation issues are discussed in Chapter 5.

The increasing role of CT in trauma is another area where radiographers have to make quick decisions about the scan protocol that will best show the diagnosis in the shortest time frame, with minimal inconvenience and discomfort to the patient. Trauma and CT are discussed within each of the relevant chapters.

Where necessary the book highlights where other modalities would be more useful, again to increase the consultancy role of the radiographer and to enable the patient to have the best possible care. This is further enhanced if radiographers undertake regular and comprehensive quality assurance (QA) tests, and act on the analysis and interpretation of the results to overcome any problems and faults demonstrated. (For more information on quality control, see Chapter 13 of Seeram's book *Computed tomography: physical principles, clinical applications and quality control*[3]). It is also important for radiographers to check that radiation doses are kept to a minimum, as it is well known that CT comprises a high proportion of medical radiation exposure and that exposure levels vary considerably between imaging departments. Adapting and optimising protocols can also have an effect on reducing CT doses, without having a significantly detrimental affect on image quality.

In order to reduce the possibility of misinterpretation, some terms have been explained and the definitions given in the CT terminology section and are used throughout the text. However, the scanner software available will depend on the equipment being utilised. Where possible the common necessities are discussed in the text. Terminology also varies between manufacturers, for example the initial planning scan may be called a scout view (IGE), topogram (Siemens) or pilot scan (Picker). These terms may vary throughout the book depending on the scanner used by each author.

Each chapter is written by a CT specialist and represents their own protocols and experience. It is hoped that their sharing of this information will make you question your own techniques and consider whether they could be improved. This book does not claim to represent the only way to undertake CT scanning.

There are many people responsible for the completion of this book; firstly all the authors, some of whom contributed at very short notice, and others who supported the venture right from the beginning. Without each and every one of those authors, this book would not have been possible.

The need for this book became apparent whilst the editor was running a CT MSc course at City University in London and found that the current available literature tended to be orientated towards physics or radiological interpretation of CT. Thanks must also go to Geoff Nuttall and Gavin Smith at GMM who believed in the project from the start and maintained that belief as time went on.

Thanks finally, to my husband, Phil, who constantly supported and encouraged me throughout the delays and always maintained I could do it.

Suzanne Henwood

References

1. College of Radiographers. *CPD facing the future together*. College of Radiographers, 1996.

2. Department of Health. *The regulations of the health professions*. Steering group chaired by Professor Sheila McClean. HMSO: London, 1996.

3. Seeram E. *Computed tomography: physical principles, clinical applications and quality control*. WB Saunders Philadelphia,. 1994.

CT TERMINOLOGY

S. Henwood, L. Donnison

Aliasing A sampling error caused by too few samples being acquired, which results in the appearance of fine lines in the final image.

Algorithm See Reconstruction algorithm.

Archival storage The storage of data for future retrieval. In currently marketed scanners the choice is 5¼ inch rewritable magneto-optical disc or digital audio tape. Other scanners may use floppy discs, 12 inch WORM (Write Once, Read Many) magneto-optical discs or large spool magnetic tape.

Artefact A representation in the image which does not originate in the object. In CT artefacts come from the patient, the CT process and the equipment.

Back projection A mathematical procedure used to reconstruct the image.

Beam hardening artefact The process of filtration of a polychromatic beam by the preferential absorption of lower energy photons, resulting in an increased effective energy. It manifests itself as dark bands or streaks in the image.

Calibration The process varies depending on the type of CT scanner used. It may include scanning air or appropriate test phantoms. Calibration takes into account variations in beam intensity or detector response in order to achieve homogeneity within the field of view and accuracy of CT number.

CT number Each picture element of the CT image is assigned a number, which corresponds to the average X-ray attenuation in that voxel. The Hounsfield scale is often utilised to represent the CT number.

Air	Water	Bone
−1000	0	+1000

Tissues more dense than water (e.g. blood and liver) have positive values and those tissues that are less dense than water (e.g. fat and lung) are given negative numbers.

The CT number can be calculated as follows:

$$\text{CT number} = \frac{\mu_t - \mu_w}{\mu_w} \times K$$

Where μ_t is the linear attenuation coefficient of the measured tissue

μ_w is the linear attenuation coefficient of water, and K is a constant, or contrast factor (In the Hounsfield Scale K = 1000, making the contrast scale 0.1% per CT number).

Collimators Depending on the system design there can be one or two sets of collimators, pre patient in the z (axis of rotation) and x (scan plane) directions and post patient in the z direction only. Collimation affects both patient dose and image quality.

Contiguous scanning Technique in non-helical scanning where two scan slices abut in order to ensure no tissue is missed.

Contrast Resolution The ability to differentiate density differences between tissues and with CT this is far superior to plain X-ray imaging. In CT this is sometimes referred to as the 'sensitivity' of the system. It is the excellent low-contrast resolution in CT which provides its superior diagnostic ability compared with plain X-rays. Low-contrast resolution is affected by photon flux, slice thickness, patient size, detector sensitivity, reconstruction algorithm, image display and recording.

CT Fluoroscopy An application of real-time CT, combining refreshed images, typically at rates of 3–6 images per second, with dynamically controlled exposures. The terminology here is vague and can mean continuous scanning with a fixed couch top position, with preprogrammed couch movement, with manual couch movement, or combined with a 'floating' couch top.

Data Acquisition The detection of transmitted X-ray photons, which are then measured and used to produce an image. Two methods are commonly used: slice by slice or volume acquisition.

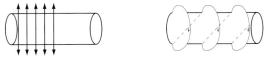
Specific slice locations   Volume scanning

Detector There are two main types of detectors, gas ionisation and scintillation. The number of detector elements varies with the type and make of scanner used. The active detectors are positioned opposite to the X-ray source, and arranged in an arc or around the circumference of the aperture. The detectors capture and convert X-ray photons into a useable signal. The more detectors per degree of arc or circumference used in each projection, the greater the resolution possible in the image.

Disc drive Stores patient information and CT scan data.

Field of View (FOV) This is the reconstruction circle, the circular region from which the transmission measurements are recorded during scanning. It is operator-selected, a smaller field of view allows better spatial resolution. On some systems the size of the field of view can affect dose.

Filter   see X-ray filter.

Fourier transform A mathematical process, which transfers a spatial domain signal into a frequency domain signal.

Gantry The gantry is the name given to the housing of the main CT scanner components (e.g. X-ray tube, detectors, motors).

Gated CT A process that uses software which synchronises the CT scanning to the patient's heart in an attempt to minimise movement unsharpness.

High-resolution CT This is used to look at fine detail. Narrow beam collimation is used to acquire slice widths down to around 1.0 mm, which reduces partial volume artefacts and improves spatial resolution. It may also be used in conjunction with a high resolution (sharp) algorithm.

Intergroup delay The time interval between two volume sequences, which allows the patient time to breathe.

Matrix The matrix is composed of pixels (or picture elements) arranged in rows and columns. The more pixels (or the larger the matrix size) the better the quality of the image.

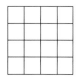

4 × 4 matrix

Common matrix sizes are
256 × 256, 320 × 320 and 512 × 512

Modulation transfer function (MTF) This is the amplitude of the output signal as a percentage of the amplitude of the input signal. The percentage amplitude is plotted against spatial frequency stated in terms of line pairs per centimetre.

Monitor Resolution A measure of the detail shown on the cathode ray tube or TV monitor. The resolution is related to the size of the pixel matrix. The display matrix is normally 512^2 (512×512) or 1024^2. High-performance monitors are available with a matrix of 2048^2, but they are not in common use.

Motion artefact Can be due to voluntary or involuntary movement of the patient and is represented by streaks on the image.

Multiplanar (MP) reconstruction Where a computer software package creates coronal, sagittal and oblique and shaped/contour images from transverse axial scans. The detail is affected predominantly by patient movement, slice thickness and the reconstruction interval in helical scanning.

Noise   Refers to the variation in CT numbers between points, when scanning a uniform object. Noise is measured by scanning a water phantom and calculating a standard deviation for a region of interest. Noise in CT is affected by the number of detected photons, slice thickness, algorithm, detector noise and object size.

Optical disc Stores data which is written and read using a laser beam. There are three basic types: CD-ROM (compact disc, read-only memory), WORM (write once, read many) and erasable optical discs.

Partial volume effect An artefact that occurs when two different densities are located within one voxel and the average of the two is displayed on the screen. This can lead to objects with small density differences being 'missed'.

Pitch Factor (often abbreviated to Pitch)

$$\frac{\text{Couch top speed (mm/s)} \times \text{tube rotation time (s)}}{\text{Nominal slice width (mm)}}$$

Pixel The pixel is the individual square picture element that makes up the matrix. The pixel is two dimensional:

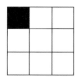

The pixel size is generally between 0.1 and 1 mm and its size can be determined as follows:

$$\text{Pixel size} = \frac{\text{Field of View (mm)}}{\text{Matrix size}}$$

Quantitative CT (QCT) Uses the numerical CT values to make a diagnosis. The term is used in particular when referring to the assessment of demineralisation in trabecular bone.

'Real time' reconstruction Generally used to describe where the reconstruction time is equal to or less than the tube/gantry rotation time. The images are either composed of 360 degrees of fresh data with one frame per rotation, or use refreshed images at varying numbers of frames per second,

Reconstruction algorithm Mathematical function that is used to enhance or suppress parts of the data. Modern scanners have several algorithms to choose from, depending on the preferred image quality.

Ring artefacts These are characteristic of third-generation scanners and are due to miscalibrated or defective detectors.

Slice thickness The thickness in the z direction of the volume being imaged. A thinner slice will give fewer streak artefacts from the partial volume effect.

Spatial resolution The ability to represent small structures. It defines the detail shown in an image. The spatial resolution of CT is much more detailed than conventional X-ray film. The MTF can be used to describe the spatial resolution of a CT system.

Voxel A three-dimensional volume element of the picture.

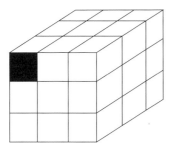

Windowing A process of manipulating the grey scale image using the CT numbers. Windowing is used by the radiographer to optimise visualisation of an image. It is the contrast of the image that is being manipulated.

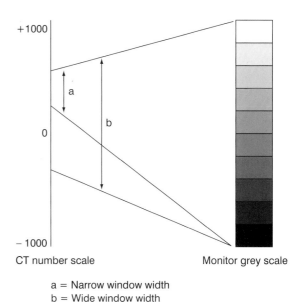

a = Narrow window width
b = Wide window width

The attenuation value scale (CT number or HU number) covers a range of about −1000 to +1000. The entire grey range is always displayed in an image but, as the human eye can only differentiate approximately 40 shades of grey, only part of the full CT number scale is selected for viewing. The **window level** is the central point of the range of CT numbers selected and the **window width** is the range of CT numbers over which the grey range is to be displayed.

X-ray Filter A filter is used to remove the unwanted soft radiation that contributes unnecessary radiation dose to the patient. Most scanners also have a shaped filter which alters the X-ray beam intensity across the field of view to take account of the reduced absorption of the beam at the periphery. The filter is usually selected automatically.

Acknowledgements

Maria Lewis, ImPACT, St George's Hospital

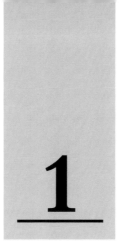

INTRODUCTION

Leigh Donnison
Suzanne Henwood

Helical scanning is a means of producing computed tomography (CT) images by combining continuous rotation of the X-ray tube around the patient with a continuously moving couch to produce an integral volume of data. Siemens were the first to market a helical scanner in 1990, quickly followed by the other CT manufacturers, and now all scanners marketed have some level of helical capability. The terms 'spiral', 'helical' or 'volume' are synonymous as far as CT terminology is concerned and vary according to the manufacturer.

There are currently nearly 370 X-ray CT scanners in use in the UK; approximately one scanner per 160 000 of the population. All the CT scanners installed since 1995, and nearly 50% of the total number of scanners, have helical capability.

In 1989, when there were just 200 working scanners in the UK, the National Radiological Protection Board (NRPB) found that CT contributed to 20% of the radiation dose due to medical radiation in diagnostic practice in the UK, although it contributed only 2% of the imaging workload. As well as the above mentioned increase in the number of scanners, the introduction of slip-ring technology has improved the capabilities of X-ray CT scanners, and allowed greater patient throughput, a greater variety of scans, and more types of investigation. It would not be unrealistic therefore to expect that the proportion of the medical radiation dose due to CT has increased.

However much manufacturers look towards dose reduction in their development programmes it is possible, even with a dose efficient system, to use an unnecessarily high mAs value. In CT scanning the user is generally rewarded for his or her mistake with a 'good' image, in contrast to other radiographic fields where overexposure results in a 'bad' film. The 1989 NRPB CT survey[1] found that for the same examination on the same scanner the mAs setting, and therefore the dose, varied by a factor of up to three. Other local examination techniques affecting the volume scanned, such as the number and width of slices and the couch increment, could vary the effective dose by factors of 5 to 20.

All of today's CT scanners have user-friendly software. Designed for a wide international market, the systems can be operated on many skill levels from 'button pushing' to employing a full understanding of CT techniques and technology. Because of the flexibility of the systems it is in the hands of the operator to use each system to its optimum.

It is in this climate of increasing CT capability and capacity that this book has been produced. Its aim is to provide the knowledge required for radiographers to adapt imaging protocols in CT. Commonly presented pathologies are used to show how scan quality can be optimised. A working knowledge of CT technology is assumed. If you require a revision of the principles of CT scanners see Seeram,[2] Webb[3] or Chiu *et al.*[4]

The first CT images produced in 1972 were crude when compared to the image quality of today's scanners, and although it is now possible to demonstrate clear grey/white matter differentiation on routine scanning, it should be remembered that before the introduction of CT scanning there was no method of imaging the brain tissue itself. Traumatic invasive procedures such as air encephalography and cerebral angiography were used to demonstrate the ventricles and vessels. These were time consuming, highly specialised procedures performed at a few specialist centres. These procedures were also were very distressing for the patient, and had a high morbidity rate. In contrast with CT scanning which is possible, as a simple outpatient procedure, to show not only the ventricles but also the soft tissues within the cranium.

As scanners developed, shorter scan times and larger X-ray tubes meant that CT could be used for body scanning allowing visualisation of the soft tissues and bones. However after a positive initial impact, it is probably true to say that CT scanning was in the doldrums for a while. In the mid to late 1980s the use of magnetic resonance imaging (MRI) took off. The number of MRI installations increased rapidly, and until the introduction of helical scanning, allowing more flexibility in the type and length of examinations, it was widely thought that CT had reached the limits of its capabilities.

As mentioned earlier, helical scanning is made possible through the use of slip-ring technology. The slip-rings enable power and data to be transferred without cables, consequently allowing continuous rotation of the tube and/or detector assembly. Previously, because of the restrictions imposed by the cables, the tube and/or detectors rotated alternately clockwise and anticlockwise. The duration of the interscan delay was at least as long as the time needed for the tube assembly to brake and then reach scanning speed again, generally this was in the region of 4 – 7 seconds. Even in non-helical scanning the interscan delay can now be the same as the time taken to increment the table by one slice width, often just 1 second. This has decreased the overall scan series acquisition times and increased the percentage of 'tube on' time.

These shorter interscan delays have reduced the amount of time available for tube cooling before the next slice is performed. Additionally, minimum 360° rotation scan times of 1 second or less are not uncommon. While shorter rotation times are obviously desirable in terms of patient movement and contrast media studies, higher mA values are needed to maintain the same photon output. These faster scan techniques have placed a huge demand on X-ray tubes, with the maximum heat capacity of X-ray tubes increasing from 4 MHU in 1995 to 7 MHU in 1997. Generators have also become correspondingly larger and are now available with up to 60 kilowatt (kW) maximum output.

One of the main advantages of helical scanning is the ability to reconstruct images at intervals less than the couch top travel per X-ray tube rotation resulting in many images from one 'scan'. These overlapping images can be used to reduce partial volume effect and improve spatial resolution in both multiplanar and three-dimensional reconstructions. Another significant advantage is the elimination of the misregistration artefacts due to irregular patient breathing that can occur in non-helical scanning.

Because helical scanning can produce many more images than non-helical scanning, and because the data set often needs to be preserved for later reconstruction a large raw data storage space is required. Computer storage and archiving facilities have increased to cope with the number of images produced. Improvements in computer technology have also resulted in much more compact scanners, with only three or four components i.e. the operator's console, gantry, couch and cabinet, whereas scanners from the early 1980s had several cabinets and other components. Where low voltage transfer is used slip-ring technology also allows the generator to be located 'on-board' as part of the rotating assembly within the gantry.

Reconstruction times have also shortened considerably, times of less than 3 seconds are common and at least one company can produce a fully reconstructed image in 1 second, allowing the reconstructed image to be viewed within 2 seconds of each tube rotation in helical scanning. This method of viewing helical images as the scan progresses is known as 'Real-time' CT. The term is generally used to describe the process where the reconstruction time is equal to or less than the tube/gantry rotation time. The images are either composed of 360° of fresh data with one frame per rotation, as in the example above, or using refreshed images at varying numbers of frames per second, (currently 3 to 8). This facility has some obvious uses: helical runs can be halted when the required area has been covered; contrast medium enhancement can be monitored and the run stopped and started where appropriate.

'CT fluoroscopy' is an application of real-time CT, combining refreshed images with dynamically controlled exposures and either a moving or fixed couch top. Extra hardware is needed. Gantry and couch movement controls can be located on a pedestal within the scan room or as a joystick on the side of the couch, with the exposure switches located either on the pedestal or as a footswitch. The proposed uses for CT fluoroscopy are mainly for biopsies, other interventional procedures and joint dynamics. CT fluoroscopy can also be combined with a C arm image intensification system, either mobile or static.

Another recent introduction is contrast bolus tracking software. This monitors the CT number of an operator-defined area as contrast medium is injected, so that the scan series can be triggered to coincide with the optimum enhancement for that region. Several companies supply this software, with differing proprietary names. The software operates by setting one or several regions of interest (ROI) on a reference scan then performing a series of scans at reduced mA values as contrast medium is injected. A graph is automatically plotted and when a predetermined rise in the HU of the ROI is reached the scan series is initiated, either manually or automatically depending on the system. Optimal contrast media timings can also be obtained prospectively by using a test bolus and then plotting a time – density curve using the scanner's analysis software functions

Automatic mA modulation software has been introduced by one manufacturer with the aim of dose reduction. The mA level is reduced both as the X-ray tube rotates around the patient and as it travels along the z axis, compensating for differences in density and thickness. Pitch can also be used to reduce dose. A pitch ratio of 1.5:1 is analogous to non-helical scanning using a 10 mm slice width and 15 mm couch top increment combination. The dose is the same but without loss of data or significant change in noise; however there is some reduction in spatial resolution perpendicular to the scan plane.

For the future, the trend continues towards shorter scan and reconstruction times combined with higher capacity tubes. Scan times may however be approaching their limits because of the great forces applied to the gantry by the rotating parts, and because of the limitations imposed by the ability of the system to acquire enough readings per second to produce an image. There is much talk of more manufacturers introducing multi row detector systems, where two or more adjacent slices are acquired in one X-ray tube rotation. Increased computing capabilities are being applied to shorten reconstruction times, reduce image artefacts and improve the post processing applications.

Acknowledgments

Maria Lewis & Sue Edyvean, ImPACT.

References

1. Shrimpton PC, Hart D, Hillier MC, Wall BV, Faulkener K *NRPB Survey of CT Practice in the UK.*

2. Seeram E. *Computed tomography: physical principles, clinical applications and quality control.* Philadelphia: WB Saunders. 1994

3. Webb S. *From the watching of shadows: the origins of radiological tomography.* Bristol: Adam Hilger, Bristol. 1990

4. Chiu LC Lipacamon JD Yiu-Chiu VS. *Clinical computed tomography for the technologist.* (2nd edn). New York: Raven Press 1995

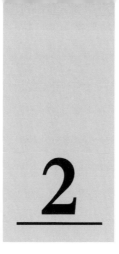

2

THE HEAD

Halina Szutowicz

Patient preparation

A simple generalised instruction leaflet is included as part of the appointment letter from the present writer's department. It includes a simple line drawing of a 'typical' CT scanner, showing that it is not enclosed or tunnel-like. There is a statement that the patient may be given an injection into one of their arm veins, and a possible waiting time of 30 minutes is also mentioned which helps the unit to cope with delays caused by emergencies.

Each patient is given an explanation of the procedure for their individual scan on being brought into the scan room. It is important to explain the need for the head rest and any immobilising straps and pads. Ensure that the patient is comfortable; use knee supports and pillows if necessary.

In the present writer's department apprehensive patients may be shown around the scanner when they come to make their appointment. This can be particularly helpful with children.

The normal CT brain scan

There is no such thing as a 'normal' brain scan; only one that is considered as normal for the age and sex of the particular subject. Figures 2.1–2.10 are scans from of a 50-year-old female whose small degree of cerebral atrophy, compatible with age, is an aid to demonstration of normal anatomy.

In the writer's unit, the preferred method of scanning is to obtain images closely compatible with those from the magnetic resonance (MR) imaging department. Most MR scans of the head are obtained using the anthropological baseline (i.e. the infraorbital meatal baseline (IOMBL)), which if used for CT would mean several scans through the eyes. The compromise is to perform routine CT of the head scanning parallel to the orbitomeatal line (radiographic baseline (RBL)) giving a variance of 12–15° of scan angle but resulting in only two sections passing through the upper orbit.

Note – unless otherwise stated all scan times are 1 second.

Note – A scan projection radiograph is not always used in the author's department.

Routine brain scan

The positions and protocols are as shown in Table 2.1.

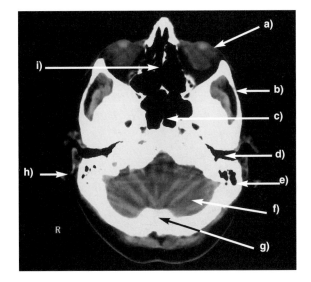

Figure 2.1 — Standard brain scan: a, orbit, note high density of the lens in the anterior aspect of the globe of the eye; b, zygomatic arch; c, sphenoid sinus; d, external auditory canal and middle ear; e, mastoid process; f, cerebellum; g, internal occipital protruberance; h, pinna of ear; i, ethmoid sinuses.

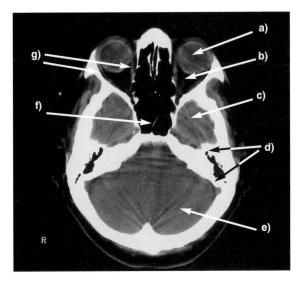

Figure 2.2 — Standard brain scan: a, globe of eye; b, optic nerve; c, temporal lobe; d, petrous temporal bone; e, cerebellum, note artefacts from internal occipital protruberance; f, sphenoid sinus; g, ocular muscles.

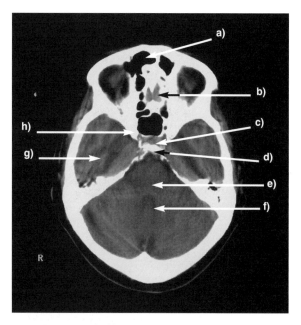

Figure 2.3 — Standard brain scan: a, frontal sinuses; b, olfactory groove; c, pituitary fossa; d, dorsum sellae; e, brain stem; f, fourth ventricle; g, temporal lobe; h, anterior clinoid process.

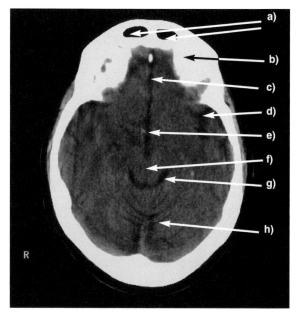

Figure 2.4 — Standard brain scan: a, frontal sinuses; b, orbital roof; c, interhemispheric fissure (anterior); d, sylvian fissure; e, third ventricle; f, midbrain; g, perimesenephalic cistons; h, cerebellar folia.

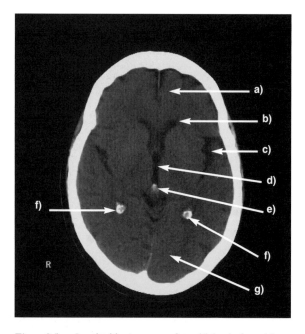

Figure 2.5 — Standard brain scan: a, frontal lobe; b, frontal horn of lateral ventricle; c, Sylvian fissure; d, third ventricle; e, pineal gland (calcified); f, choroid plexus (calcified); g, occipital lobe.

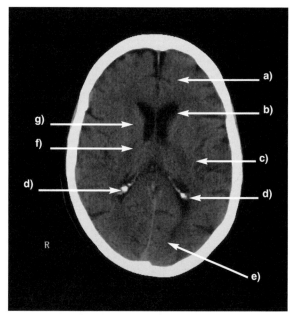

Figure 2.6 — Standard brain scan: a, frontal lobe; b, frontal horn of lateral ventricle; c, parietal lobe; d, choroid plexus; e, occipital lobe; f, internal capsule; g, caudate nucleus.

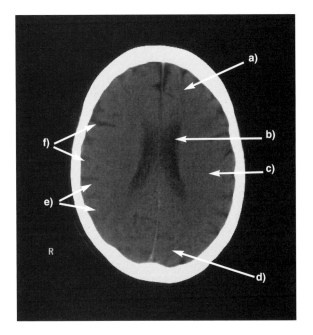

Figure 2.7 — Standard brain scan: a, frontal lobe; b, body of lateral ventricle; c, parietal lobe; d, occipital lobe; e, gyri; f, sulci.

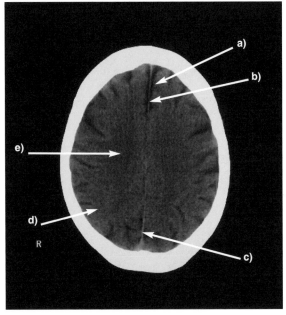

Figure 2.8 — Standard brain scan: a, interhemispheric fissure; b, anterior falx cerebri; c, posterior falx cerebri; d, grey matter; e, white matter.

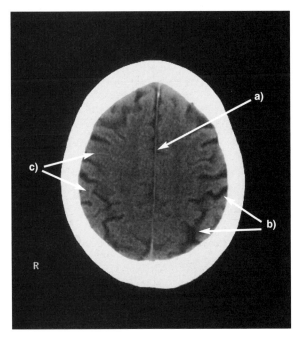

Figure 2.9 — Standard brain scan: a, falx cerebri; b, sulci; c, gyri.

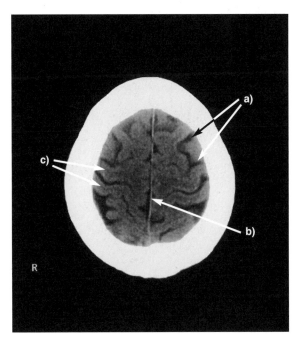

Figure 2.10 — Standard brain scan: a, sulci; b, falx cerebri; c, gyri.

Table 2.1 – Protocol for routine brain scan

Patient position	Supine, head in head rest, scanner gantry parallel to radiographic baseline (RBL). Head in centre of scan field. (Lateral scan projection radiograph may be used if required)
Start position	RBL

Protocol	
Slice thickness	10 mm
Table increment	10 mm
Kilovoltage	120 kV
mAs per slice	300 mAs
Algorithm	Standard
Scan field of view	25 cm
Display field of view	25 cm
Window width (WW)	150/100/80
Window level (WL)	40

Adapting technique to the pathology and the patient

THE POSTERIOR FOSSA

When the clinical information clearly indicates a posterior fossa or mid-brain pathology the slice width and table incrementation are adjusted to 5 mm (or in some cases 3 mm) to better demonstrate these areas. It may be necessary to adjust the mAs per slice to 320 mAs to obtain a comparable image quality. For most adults 8–10 sections will be done on average. Begin the scan 1 cm below and parallel to the RBL.

PAEDIATRICS

It is necessary to adapt techniques to suit the wide variety of child and infant sizes. Basic protocols for paediatric use are suggested in Tables 2.2–2.4.

After 7 years of age the adult programme can be used, with reduced mAs values until the child's head is approaching adult size. (Note that the skull vault will have achieved adult size before the facial bones have matured to adult proportions.)

Equally, it may be necessary to reduce mAs values for very petite adults.

Table 2.2 – Basic paediatric protocol: neonate

Patient position	Supine, head in head rest, scanner gantry parallel to RBL. Head in centre of scan field.
Start position	RBL

Protocol	
Slice thickness	7 mm
Table increment	7 mm
Kilovoltage	100 kv
mAs per slice	100 mAs
Algorithm	Soft/standard
Scans field of view	25 cm
Display field of view	20 cm
Window width	150/100/80
Window level	40

Table 2.3 – Basic paediatric protocol: 6 months–2 years

Patient position	Supine, head in head rest, scanner gantry parallel to RBL. Head in centre of scan field.
Start position	RBL

Protocol	
Slice thickness	7 mm
Table increment	7 mm
Kilovoltage	100 kv
mAs per slice	150 mAs
Algorithm	Standard
Scan field of view	25 cm
Display field of view	22 cm
Window width	150/100/80
Window level	40

Table 2.4 – Basic paediatric protocol: 2 years–7 years

Patient position	Supine, head in head rest, scanner gantry parallel to RBL. Head in centre of scan field.
Start position	RBL

Protocol	
Slice thickness	10 mm
Table increment	10 mm
Kilovoltage	120 kV
mAs per slice	200 mAs
Algorithm	Standard
Scan field of view	25 cm
Display field of view	22 cm
Window width	150/100/80
Window level	40

Contrast media usage

The policy in the present author's unit is to keep contrast usage as low as possible and it is felt that there are certain circumstances where contrast should not be used in the first instance, that is:

- early on in any situation of haemorrhage or infarction;
- in pituitary scans when the prolactin level is below 2000 units;
- in patients with a previously recorded allergic reaction to iodine;
- in inadequately prepared children.

However there are also circumstances when the unenhanced scan is dispensed with. These include:

- tumour follow-up;
- where there is a strong possibility of metastatic deposits from the clinical history;
- where the history is suggestive of acoustic neuroma (normally examined with MR);
- with pituitary lesions where prolactin levels are above 2000 units.

The dosage is shown in Table 2.5.

Table 2.5 – Dosage of contrast medium

Non-ionic contrast medium	300 mg/iodine/ml is always used
Adults	50 ml
Children	1 ml/kilogram, up to 50 kg
CT angiogram	100 ml, via 16 gauge venous cannula, connector and three-way tap. Use injection arm board.

Trauma

Presentations are widely variable and the scan must be tailored to the individual case. However some basic guidelines and protocols can be used. In some cases of multiple trauma it may not be possible to use the head rest and head immobilising pads should be available to allow scanning on the couch top.

If there is evidence of facial injury it is appropriate to perform scans of the facial skeleton at the same time, as this will assist the maxillofacial surgeon's assessment of injury. In cases of multiple trauma it may be appropriate to perform a lateral scan projection radiograph of the cervical spine to better assess the C7/T1 area (see p. 39: Fig 3.9). This should be done using high kV and

mA values to produce an image where the available information can be manipulated to produce optimal visualisation.

Head injury without facial trauma

A protocol for this situation is given in Table 2.6. Always view and image on bone settings, as well as standard brain settings, to demonstrate any bony injury.

Table 2.6 – Protocol for head injury without facial trauma

Patient position	Supine, head in head rest if possible, scanner gantry parallel to RBL. Head in centre of scan field.
Start position	Foramen Magnum

Protocol	
Slice thickness	10 mm
Table increment	10 mm
Kilovoltage	120 kV
mAs per slice	300 mAs
Algorithm	Standard
Scan field of view	25 cm
Display field of view	25 cm
Window width	150/100/80
Window level	40
Bone window width	1500
Bone window level	500

Head injury with facial trauma

Table 2.7 gives a suitable protocol. Again, one should always view and image on bone settings as well as standard brain settings to demonstrate any bony injury.

Table 2.7 – Protocol for head injury with facial trauma

Patient position	Supine, head in head rest if possible, scanner gantry parallel to infraorbital meatal baseline (IOMBL). Head in centre of scan field.
Start position	Alveolar margin of maxilla
End position	Supraorbital margin

Protocol	
Slice thickness	5 mm
Table increment	5 mm
Kilovoltage	120kV
mAs per slice	300 mAs
Algorithm	Standard
Scan field of view	25 cm
Display field of view	25 cm

Table 2.7 – continued

Window width	150/100/80
Window level	40
Bone window width	1500
Bone window level	500

Scan remaining area as trauma above, on 10 mm slice and increment.

Multiple trauma

Major trauma patients may only have had basic advanced trauma life support (ATLS) protocol radiographs (lateral cervical spine, pelvis and chest), and the difficulties in obtaining a good lateral cervical spine image are well appreciated. If the patient requires CT for other injuries, a lateral scan projection radiograph can be taken to better visualise the cervical region, especially at the cervicothoracic junction. Table 2.8 describes a protocol for this. (Page 40 Fig 3.9 illustrates the result).

Examples of scans taken from trauma patients are shown in Figures 2.11–2.13.

Table 2.8 – Lateral scan projection radiograph of the cervical region

Patient position	Supine, head in head rest if possible, scanner gantry vertical. Cervical spine centred within gantry.
Start position	5 cm above pinna of ear
End position	Sternal angle
Protocol	
Table movement	30 cm
Kilovoltage	140 kV
mA	200–400 mA
Algorithm	Standard
X-ray tube position	Lateral
Window width	Choose suitable levels
Window level	to demonstrate each area of cervical spine

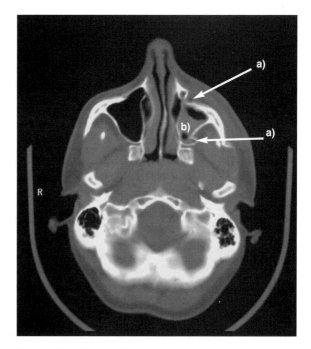

Figure 2.11 — Trauma, 5 mm axial facial scan on bone windows: a, fractures of maxillary antrum (arrowed); b, fluid within maxillary antrum.

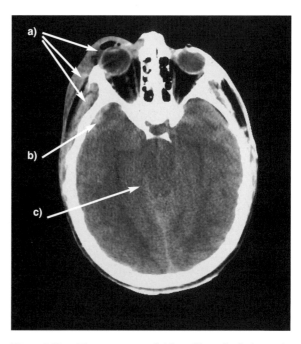

Figure 2.12 — Trauma: a, superficial swelling of soft tissues; b, contusion in temporal lobe; c, perimesencephalic cistons not visible (indicates raised intracranial pressure).

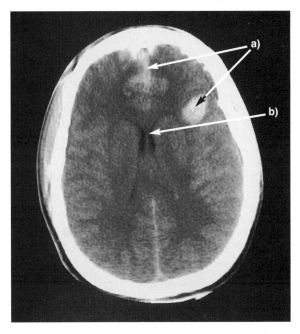

Figure 2.13 — Trauma: a, intracerebral contusions; b, small ventricles (indicates raised intracranial pressure.

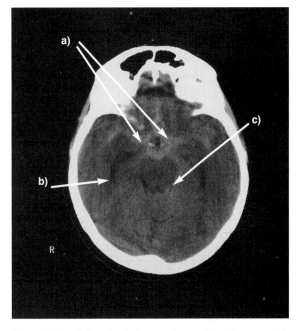

Figure 2.14 — Subarachnoid haemorrhage: a, blood in suprasellar cisterns; b, dilation of temporal horns of lateral ventricles (early hydrocephalus); c, blood in permesencephalic cistons.

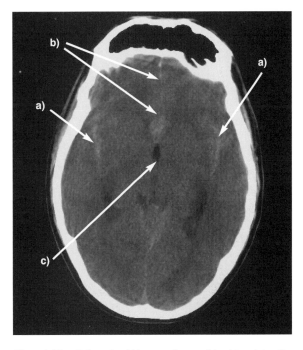

Figure 2.15 — Subarachnoid haemorrhage: a, blood in sylvian fissures bilaterally; b, blood in interhemisphere fissure anteriorly; c, prominence of third ventricle (early hydrocephalus).

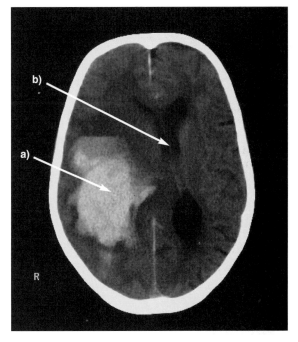

Figure 2.16 — Intracerebral haemorrhage: a, massive right parietal haematoma; b, midline shift and ventricular compression.

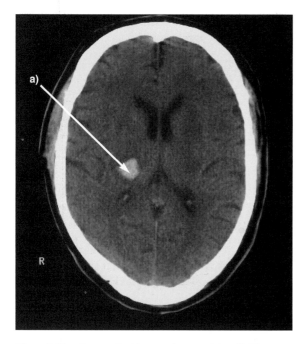

Figure 2.17 — Intracerebral haemorrhage: a, right-sided haemor-rhage within the internal capsule. The site of the haemorrhage will result in a dense left hemiplegia despite the small size of the haematoma.

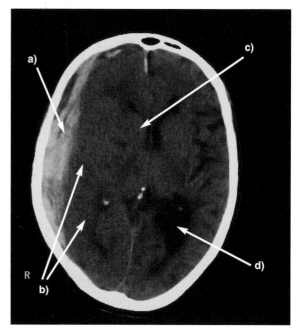

Figure 2.18 — Acute subdural haematoma: a, concave shape to edge of haematoma; b, effacement of sulci on affected side; c, midline shift and compression of ipsilateral ventricle; d, dilation of contralateral ventricle.

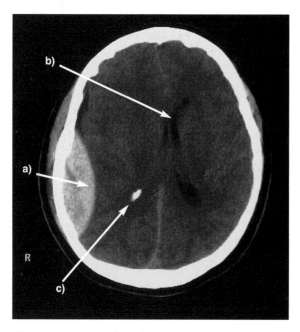

Figure 2.19 — Extradural haematoma: a, convex shape of haematoma; b, ventricular compression and midline shift; c, ele-vation of right choroid plexus.

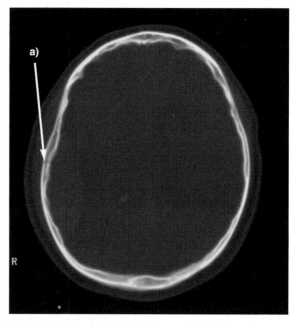

Figure 2.20 — Extradural haematoma: a, skull fracture underlying haematoma seen on bone windows.

Haemorrhage

Acute haemorrhage

Scans for spontaneous subarachnoid haemorrhage (Figures 2.14 and 2.15) or intracerebral haemorrhage (Figures 2.16 and 2.17), as well as for acute traumatic subdural (Figure 2.18) and extradural (Figures 2.19 and 2.20) haematomas are all most likely to be undertaken as emergency procedures. All these conditions have dramatically different and diagnostic appearances in most cases, although in trauma it is possible to have combinations of some or all of the types.

SCANNING PROTOCOL FOR ACUTE HAEMORRHAGE

A routine brain scanning protocol (see p. 12) is used. Posterior fossa haemorrhages are a very small proportion of these presentations and if necessary they can be clarified with narrow slice imaging later. Note that no contrast medium whatsoever should be administered in the acute phase.

Most subarachnoid haemorrhage and some intracerebral haemorrhage patients will undergo diagnostic cerebral angiography to clarify the findings of the CT scan and prior to possible surgery, or endovascular embolisation.

Chronic subdural haematoma
(Figures 2.21 and 2.22)

This is not an emergency situation as the patients frequently present days or whole weeks following a relatively trivial injury. The patients are typically elderly and have a history of slow onset of neurological disorder, but an accurate history is important to establish the timescale, as the age of the subdural haematoma will determine the CT appearance.

SCANNING PROTOCOL FOR CHRONIC SUBDURAL HAEMATOMA

A routine brain scanning protocol is used (see p. 12). Contrast medium enhancement may be useful in some cases of isodense subdural haematoma, but most modern scanners will produce image quality that will distinguish the brain edge from the isodense haematoma. Contrast enhancement will make this interface more obvious.

Infarction

Cerebral infarction presents in many different ways and it may be of some use to clarify some of the terminology used when requests are made (Box 2.1). Strictly speaking, a cerebral infarct is not an indication for an emergency scan, but the need to begin anticoagulant

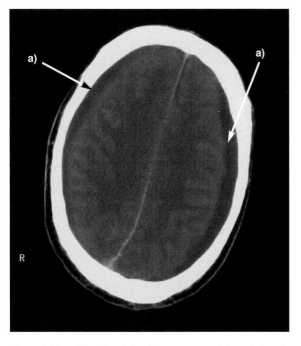

Figure 2.21 — Chronic subdural haematoma: a, bilateral chronic subdural collections, the left being larger than the right.

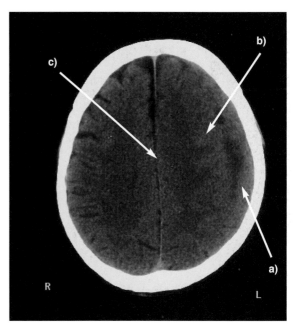

Figure 2.22 — Isodense subdural haematoma: a, isodense subdural collection; b, compressed cortex, effacement of cerebral sulci; c, minimal midline shift.

treatment often means that a scan as soon as feasible will distinguish between a haemorrhage and an infarction. The CT scan appearances of infarction may not be evident for 48–72 hours except in the rare situation of infarction of the whole hemisphere or of one of the major cerebral vessels.

Scanning protocol for cerebral infarction
(Figures 2.23–2.26)

A routine brain scanning protocol is used (see p. 12). Contrast medium is not required.

Appearance of scan

Scans performed more than 72 hours after an infarction with incomplete neurological recovery will reveal changes, and in patients who have had several episodes of TIA or RIND it may also be possible to demonstrate small areas of infarction. There are several features which distinguish infarction from other diagnoses.

- It involves both grey and white matter.
- It is non-space occupying (except when involving major vessel infarction, when there will be some oedema).
- Typical 'wedge-shaped' area of tissue loss.

Box 2.1	CEREBROVASCULAR CONDITIONS: SOME TERMINOLOGY
Stroke	Can mean either a haemorrhage or a thrombosis.
Infarction	Damage to an area of the brain, caused by permanent loss of the blood supply. Presentation will usually be that of a sudden onset of neurological deficit which may improve to some degree with time as collateral circulation is established.
TIA	Transient ischaemic attack. Temporary loss of blood supply to either the whole or part of one cerebral hemisphere as a result of narrowing of the carotid artery in the neck. The duration of a TIA can be from minutes to some hours but resolves with full restoration of function.
Amaurosis fugax	TIA in the blood supply to the eye resulting in temporary blindness in one eye.
RIND	Reversible ischaemic neurological deficit. Similar in nature to a transient ischaemic attack but lasts for up to 24 hours and then recovers.

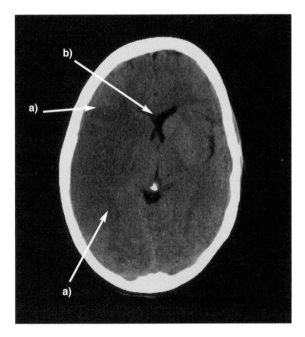

Figure 2.23 — Infarction. Right middle cerebral artery infarct: a, wedge-shaped low density area involving both grey and white matter; b, some midline shift and compression of the lateral ventricle.

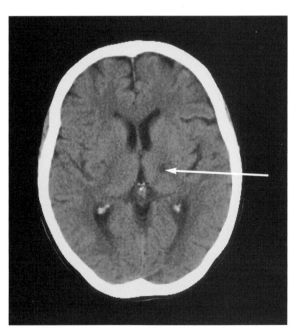

Figure 2.24 — Infarction: lacuna infarct arrowed.

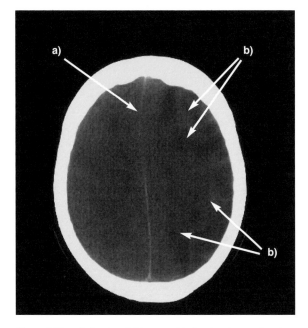

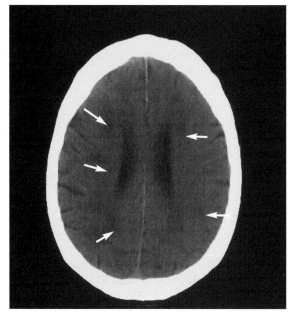

Figure 2.25 — Infarction. Major vessel infarction (acute phase): a, midline shift; b, extensive low density areas involving both grey and white matter.

Figure 2.26 — Infarction. Multi-infarct disease: many small areas of infarction (arrowed).

- Local dilation of cerebrospinal fluid pathways replacing destroyed brain tissues.

Tumours

It is not within the scope of this chapter to cover the multitude of tumour presentations for CT scanning. Whole books have been devoted to the CT appearances of brain tumours and the reader can refer to these for detailed information. Some typical features of presentation and scan appearances for two main classifications of brain tumours, malignant and benign, are presented here.

Malignant tumours (Figures 2.27–2.29)

It should be remembered that the most common example of any brain neoplasm encountered will be a secondary deposit from another primary source. The general term 'glioma' covers a range of primary malignant brain tumours with a wide variation in histological appearance. Malignant brain tumours invade normal brain tissue and often grow rapidly, causing reactive oedema around the affected area and increasing the mass effect of the lesion. There is a wide variety of brain malignancies which present in childhood.

Indications – These include presentation with neurological signs of a progressive nature, usually of short dura-tion, with or without a history of a primary lesion elsewhere, and no possibility of a vascular cause.

Scanning protocol – A routine brain scan protocol is employed, before and after administration of 50ml of contrast medium.

Follow up – A routine brain protocol is used, after contrast injection.

Benign tumours

These tumours are non-aggressive and will be slow-growing, compressing normal brain tissue rather than invading it. Neurological signs may be very slow to become noticeable as the brain will compensate for the slow compression over time. Examples are meningioma (Figures 2.30 and 2.31), craniopharyngioma and acoustic neuroma (see posterior fossa tumours, p. 21) Slow-growing tumours frequently have calcification within them.

Scanning protocol – Routine brain scanning protocol is used before and after contrast administration.

Follow up – If calcification is demonstrated in the original scan, pre and post contrast scans should be performed. If no calcification is present, a contrast-enhanced scan only is performed.

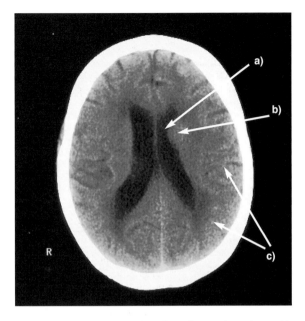

Figure 2.27 — Tumours. Unenhanced scan in patient with known primary carcinoma: a, compression of left lateral ventricle; b, possible area of increased attenuation; c, effacement of sulci in left hemisphere.

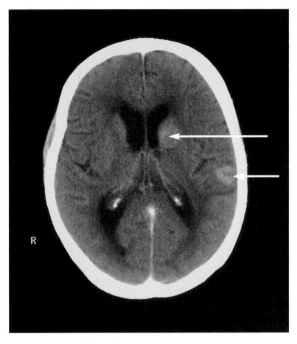

Figure 2.28 — Tumours. The same patient as in Figure 2.27, post contrast enhancement. Metastatic deposits are arrowed. There were multiple small metastatic lesions throughout the brain.

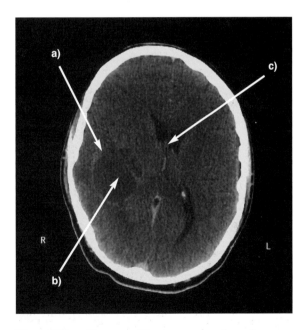

Figure 2.29 — Tumours. Glioma, contrast-enhanced scan: a, irregular enhancing tumour wall; b, cystic loculated necrotic centre; c, midline shift. Note: the patient was already on steroid treatment which has reduced the reactive white matter oedema.

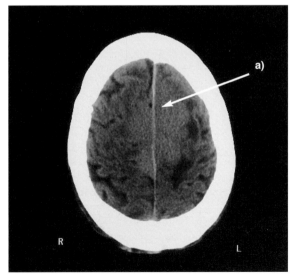

Figure 2.30 — Benign tumours. Parafalcine meningioma, unenhanced scan: a, homogeneous tissue, slightly increased attenuation.

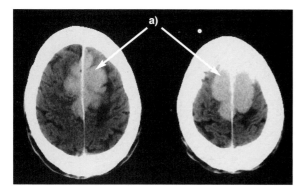

Figure 2.31 — Benign tumours. Parafalcine meningioma, post contrast enhancement: a, tumour enhances evenly.

Posterior fossa tumours (Figures 2.32 and 2.33)

The posterior fossa is best examined by magnetic resonance imaging whenever possible; however it is necessary to have specific protocols available when MR is not available, or as an option for particular patients. CT is often essential for the demonstration and assessment of skull base lesions, such as chordoma or glomus jugularae tumours.

Patients will present with symptoms of posterior fossa neurology, ataxia, giddiness, hearing loss, lower cranial nerve palsies and, if metastatic disease is suspected, a history of a primary lesion elsewhere.

Table 2.9 describes a standard protocol for scanning the posterior fossa.

Table 2.9 – Standard posterior fossa scanning protocol

Patient position	Supine, head in head rest, scanner gantry parallel to IOMBL. Head in centre of scan field.
Start position	Foramen magnum (lateral scan projection radiograph is optional)
End position	3rd ventricle

Protocol	
Slice thickness	5 mm
Table increment	5 mm
Kilovoltage	120 kV
mAs per slice	320 mAs
Algorithm	Standard
Scan field of view	25 cm
Display field of view	25 cm
Window width	200/150
Window level	40

Scan the remainder of the head in 10 mm slices and increments.

Pre and post contrast studies should be performed. On occasion it may be necessary to use narrower slice widths (e.g. 3 mm) to better demonstrate some lesions. The small vascular nodules of the haemangiomas characteristic of Von Hippel–Lindau disease are a good example of a case where narrower slice thickness may be required.

Acoustic neuroma

A scan protocol for this condition is given in Table 2.10.

Table 2.10 – Protocol for acoustic neuroma

Scanning protocol	Routine posterior fossa scan protocol as above following contrast injection. Identify the precise location of the internal auditory meatus from these scans and repeat scans, 1 mm slice thickness and 1 mm intervals, to image through the meatus. Use a smaller display field of view, 15 cm, (if available) and image on both soft tissue and bone algorithms.

Soft tissue	
Window width	200/150/120
Window level	40
Bone	
Window width	4000/1500
Window level	800/250

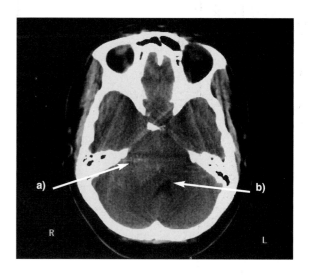

Figure 2.32 — Posterior fossa. Petrous ridge meningioma: a, area of increased attenuation with flecks of calcification; b, distortion and shift from midline of fourth ventricle.

Skull base tumours

CT imaging of the bone erosion or destruction of skull base tumours is needed as an adjunct to MRI. Table 2.11 describes the protocol.

Table 2.11 – Skull base scanning protocol

A LATERAL SCAN PROJECTION RADIOGRAPH SHOULD BE PERFORMED	
Start position	1 cm below formen magnum
End position	Upper border of petrous bone
Gantry angle	Parallel to posterior fossa skull base
Protocol	
Slice thickness	3 mm
Table increment	3 mm
Kilovoltage	120 kV
mAs per slice	200 mAs
Algorithm	Bone/edge
Scan field of view	25 cm
Display field of view	20 cm
Window width	4000/2000/15000
Window level	800/400/250

If MR imaging has not been performed it will be necessary to perform the CT scan with contrast and use a higher mAs setting; this is in order to post process into a soft tissue or standard algorithm to assess the soft tissue component of these types of lesion (Figure 2.34).

Pituitary fossa lesions

These are best examined by MR imaging, but if CT is to be used then coronal images are essential. Direct coronal imaging is obviously the best method but thin slice axial images and post processing to the coronal plane can be satisfactory. Table 2.12 gives the protocol (Figures 2.35–2.36).

The thin slices will allow a sagittal reformat if needed. Contrast medium is used if prolactin levels are above 2000 units.

Infection (Figures 2.37–39)

Cerebral abscess is a very rare condition and is almost always associated with concurrent infection in the paranasal sinuses or mastoid bones, leading to abscess formation in the frontal lobes, temporal lobes or posterior fossa. Abscess formation in other sites is either due to injury or surgery or, very rarely, caused by septic emboli in a patient with a pre-existing cardiac anomaly. Even rarer than a discrete abscess cavity is the subdural or extradural empyema where the infection tracks along the subdural space or forms between the bone and the dura.

Table 2.12 – Protocol for pituitary fossa lesions

Patient position	Prone, head in head rest with chin extended and elevated on small positioning pads. Perform a lateral scan projection radiograph.
Start position	Anterior clinoid processes/ planum sphenoidale
End position	Posterior clinoid processes/ dorsum sella
Gantry angle	90° to floor of pituitary fossa
Protocol	
Slice thickness	1 mm
Table increment	1 mm
Kilovoltage	120 kV
mAs per slice	320 mAs
Algorithm	Detail
Scan field of view	25 cm
Display field of view	17 cm
Window width	400
Window level	20

Reverse the image to display in the anatomical position

Prior to the formation of a discrete abscess cavity, the affected area of brain is described as having cerebritis, an area of infection within the brain tissue. This will be oedematous and will have generalised patchy enhancement following intravenous contrast medium injection. See Figures 2.37 and 2.38.

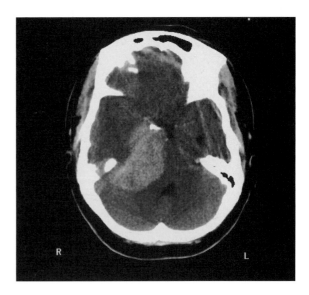

Figure 2.33 — Posterior fossa. Petrous ridge meningioma, post contrast enhancement.

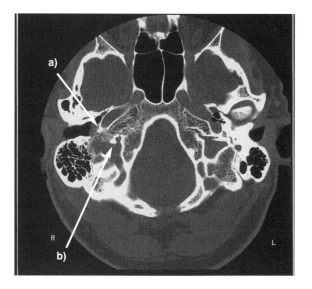

Figure 2.34 — Posterior fossa, skull base. Glomus jugularae tumour: a, soft tissue component in middle ear cavity; b, erosion of margins of jugular foramen in skull base.

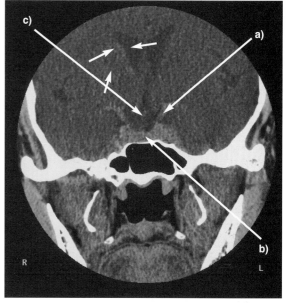

Figure 2.35 — Pituitary fossa. Contrast-enhanced coronal scan: a, internal carotid artery; b, normal pituitary gland; c, pituitary stalk.

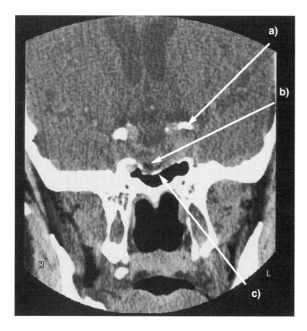

Figure 2.36 — Pituitary fossa. Coronal scan, contrast-enhanced, of pituitary adenoma: a, anterior clinoid process; b, low density tumour within pituitary gland; c, depression and erosion of floor of pituitary fossa.

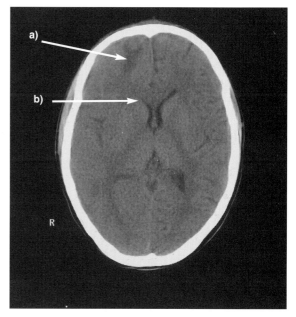

Figure 2.37 — Intracranial infection. Right frontal cerebritis, unenhanced; a, area of low attenuation; b, compression of right frontal horn.

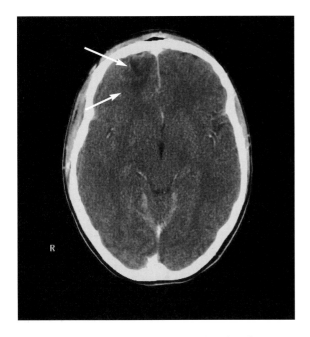

Figure 2.38 — Intracranial infection. Right frontal cerebritis, contrast-enhanced. Note enhancement around low density area (arrows).

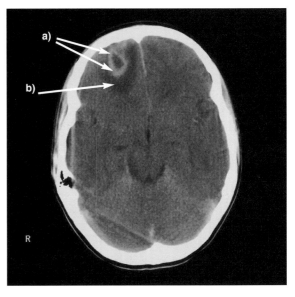

Figure 2.39 — Intracranial infection. Same patient as in Figure 2.38. 3 days later. Contrast-enhanced right frontal cerebral abscess: a, thick, irregular enhancing wall; b, surrounding reactive oedema.

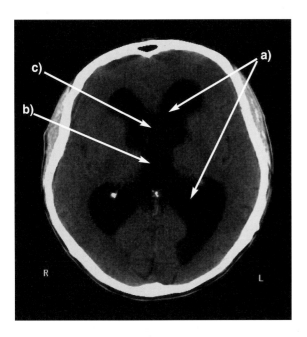

Figure 2.40 — Hydrocephalus: a, dilated lateral ventricles; b, dilated third ventricle; c, cavum septum pellucidum (a normal variant).

Scanning of patients with suspected meningitis is a common request for two main reasons:

1) to exclude the possibility of subarachnoid haemorrhage due to the similarity of some of the presenting symptoms;

2) to establish that there is no raised intracranial pressure prior to diagnostic lumbar puncture.

Scanning protocol for cerebral infection

It is emphasised that all cases of cerebral infection must have an initial unenhanced scan. If this is entirely normal (as in most cases of meningitis) then this scan will be sufficient. All scans with abnormal appearances will require contrast enhancement. Cerebral infection will normally involve large amounts of reactive oedema and space occupation, and the patients will be very seriously ill, usually pyrexial and have marked neurological deficit. As previously stated these patients will also have some history of a source of a related infection in the sinuses or mastoids.

The routine brain scanning protocol should be used or if the abscess is in the posterior fossa 5mm sections should be performed through the relevant area.

Follow up – Contrast-enhanced scans only are required.

Hydrocephalus (Figure 2.40)

Whilst hydrocephalus may be an incidental finding on a routine scan, most scanning for hydrocephalus will be performed as routine assessment or monitoring in patients with ventricular shunts. With the use of newer adjustable pressure systems, these patients are likely to have a large number of examinations in their lifetime, and it is important to establish a low-dose limited protocol to reduce the radiation burden in these cases.

Scanning protocol for hydrocephalus

As the request is usually to demonstrate ventricular size, the protocol described in Table 2.13 is recommended. A lateral scan projection radiograph should be used.

Only five or six sections will be taken, reducing the dose to the patient by at least half as the mAs used is also substantially reduced.

Table 2.13 – Scanning protocol for hydrocephalus

PERFORM A LATERAL SCAN PROJECTION RADIOGRAPH	
Patient position	Supine with head in head rest
Start position	1 cm above orbital roof
End position	Skull vault
Gantry angle	Parallel to RBL
Protocol	
Slice thickness	10 mm
Table increment	20 mm
Kilovoltage	120 kV
mAs per slice	200 mAs
Algorithm	Standard
Scan field of view	25 cm
Display field of view	25 cm
Window width	100/80
Window level	40

Vascular studies (Figure 2.41)

Indications

1. To identify aneurysms of the Circle of Willis in patients presenting without a subarachnoid haemorrhage. Examples are 3rd and 6th cranial nerve palsies often accompanied by pain. The protocol is also used in very elderly patients presenting with subarachnoid haemorrhage, when formal angiography may not be a serious option but a diagnosis is needed.

2. Visualisation of arteriovenous malformations in 3D format in conjunction with formal angiography to plan surgery or endovascular treatment.

SCANNER REQUIREMENTS

Continuous volume scanning mode (helical/spiral) and a 3D post processing software package are essential. Desirable features would include an 'intelligent' scan start function which automatically starts the scan at maximum contrast enhancement.

SCANNING PROTOCOL FOR ANEURYSM

A lateral scan projection radiograph must be performed. Details of the protocol are given in Table 2.14.

Table 2.14 – Protocol for aneurysm

PERFORM A LATERAL SCAN PROJECTION RADIOGRAPH	
Patient position	Supine with head in head rest
Start position	Half-way between pituitary fossa floor and anterior clinoid processes.
End position	30 mm above start position.
Gantry angle	Parallel to radiographic baseline
Protocol	
Slice thickness	1 mm
Table increment (pitch)	1 mm
Kilovoltage	120 kV
mAs per slice	280–300 mAs
Algorithm	Standard
Scan field of view	25 cm
Display field of view	18 cm
Window width	200
Window level	40
Scan start delay (average)	15 sec

Contrast injection is via a large gauge venous cannula, a connector and a three-way tap. A volume of 100 ml of contrast medium is injected, and scanning commences after the predetermined delay time to allow scans to be taken during the 'first pass' of contrast through the Circle of Willis. The delay time is varied to suit the age of the patient. (The 'intelligent start' feature of some scanners, mentioned above, would be appropriate in this situation.)

SCANNING PROTOCOL FOR ARTERIOVENOUS MALFORMATION

Scans may have to be obtained with a wider slice and table increment (pitch of 1) 3 mm or 5 mm and post

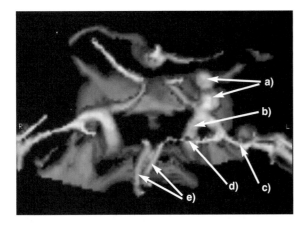

Figure 2.41 — Vascular studies. 3D reconstruction of CT angiogram of Circle of Willis viewed from anterosuperiorly: a, biloculated posterior communicating artery aneurysm; b, internal carotid artery; c, middle cerebral artery; d, anterior cerebral artery; e, pericallosal arteries.

processed into 1mm increments to produce a smoother 3D reconstruction. Otherwise the protocol is the same as for aneurysms, with the exception of the position which would have to be selected according to the location of the lesion.

Vascular studies can also be performed in the neck to demonstrate the carotid bifurcation in carotid artery stenosis. Again protocol adaptations will need to be made to cover the appropriate area. Pre contrast studies in the neck will be useful in locating the correct levels to scan and also to identify any calcification in the arterial walls. The start delay time of the scan will be adjusted by a few seconds to scan during the 'first pass' of contrast in the neck.

Neck and postnasal space

It is not intended to include full explanations of scanning of the neck but only of those procedures commonly required of a neuroradiological scanner.

Postnasal space

The usual indications are for the diagnosis and monitoring of tumours of the postnasal space. Contrast enhancement is not usually necessary as the loss of tissue planes and bone erosion or deformity are well demonstrated in axial sections.

SCANNING PROTOCOL FOR POSTNASAL SPACE

Lateral scan projection radiograph is optional. The details are given in Table 2.15.

Table 2.15 – Protocol for postnasal space scan

Patient position	Supine with head in head cushion on table top
Start position	Skull base
End position	Epiglottis
Gantry angle	Parallel to infraorbital meatal line
Protocol	
Slice thickness	5 mm
Table increment	5 mm
Kilovoltage	120 kV
mAs per slice	250 mAs
Algorithm	Soft/standard
Scan field of view	25 cm
Display field of view	22 cm
Window width	400
Window level	20

Salivary glands

Examination of salivary masses is performed both before and after contrast enhancement. Involvement of and delineation of the site of the carotid arteries and jugular veins is essential when surgery is being considered (Figure 2.42).

SCANNING PROTOCOL FOR PAROTID OR SUBMANDIBULAR GLANDS

This is described in Table 2.16. A lateral scan projection radiograph is essential.

The scans should then be repeated following injection of 50 ml of contrast medium, beginning at the end of the injection and scanning in a cranial direction to benefit from the arterial directional flow.

Sinuses (Figures 2.43 and 2.44)

It is currently accepted that the best assessment of the paranasal sinuses is CT scanning in the coronal plane. Otolaryngologists routinely perform fibreoptic endoscopic examination and surgery (FESS) in the sinuses and will require CT assessment in the manner that is closest to the way the sinuses will be visualised at surgery.

Table 2.16 – Protocol for parotid or submandibular glands

PERFORM A LATERAL SCAN PROJECTION RADIOGRAPH

Patient position	Supine with head in head cushion on table top
Start position	Supraorbital margin (parotid) External auditory meatus (submandibular)
End position	Cervical vertebra or lower extent of mass
Gantry angle	Parallel to infraorbital meatal line

Protocol	
Slice thickness	5 mm
Table increment	5 mm
Kilovoltage	120 kV
mAs per slice	250 mAs
Algorithm	Soft/standard
Scan field of view	25 cm
Display field of view	18/20 cm
Window width	300/400
Window level	20/40

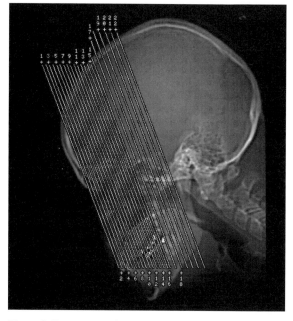

Figure 2.43 — Paranasal sinuses. Lateral scan projection radiograph shows cut lines for routine scan protocol.

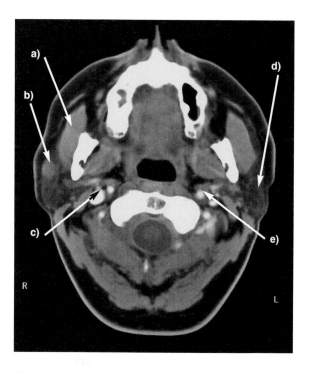

Figure 2.42 — Contrast-enhanced scan for right parotid mass: a, masseter muscle; b, enhancing nodule in right parotid gland; c, right jugular vein; d, normal left parotid gland; e, left internal carotid artery.

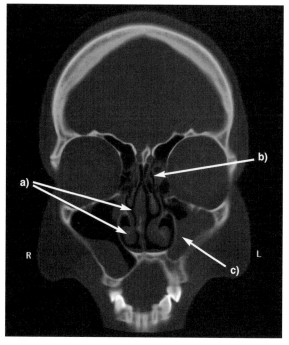

Figure 2.44 — Paranasal sinuses. Coronal section: a, mucosal thickening in nasal cavity; b, mucosal thickening in ethmoid sinuses; c, mucosal thickening in maxillary sinuses.

Scanning protocol for coronal projection of sinuses

Lateral scan projection radiograph is essential. Details are given in Table 2.17.

Table 2.17 – Protocol for coronal projection of sinuses

PERFORM A LATERAL SCAN PROJECTION RADIOGRAPH	
Patient position	Prone with head extended and chin supported on additional pads in the head rest
Start position	Anterior margin of frontal sinus
End position	Posterior wall of sphenoid sinus
Gantry angle	Parallel to posterior wall of maxillary sinus and at 90° to hard palate
Protocol	
Slice thickness	3 or 5 mm
Table increment	3 or 5 mm
Kilovoltage	120 kV
mAs per slice	150 or 200 mAs
Algorithm	Bone or detail
Scan field of view	25 cm
Display field of view	20 cm
Window width	4000
Window level	800/700

3 mm scans and increment from frontal sinus to posterior wall of maxillary sinus, and 5 mm scans and increment for the remainder.

Comments

Imaging should be done with a right–left reverse to image in the anatomical position, and the recommended window settings will demonstrate both bone margins and soft tissue content in the sinuses, whilst minimising artefacts from dental fillings and bridges. Low mA values can be used as the imaging is primarily of bony margins and air spaces. Prone coronal imaging is preferable to head-hanging supine coronal imaging as patient immobilisation is much better.

Supplementary techniques

Axial imaging – using scanning factors and algorithms similar to the coronal protocol, may sometimes be required to fully delineate tumours and is essential in the evaluation of Wegener's granuloma. If coronal images have been obtained, a 5 mm slice width and increment is adequate for the axial images. If however coronal positioning has been impossible, axial images should be obtained at 3 mm slice and increment, from the alveolar process of the maxilla to the upper limit of the frontal sinus, with a gantry angle parallel to the RBL.

Orbits

Indications

Scanning of the orbit is required for a wide variety of conditions including thyroid eye disease, orbital and retro-orbital tumours, lacrimal gland tumours, periorbital infections, intraocular foreign bodies and angular dermoids.

Techniques

There are several variations on the techniques involved, to suit the clinical presentation.

Patient positioning in the axial and coronal planes is the same as for sinuses. Gantry angulations are as follows.

- *Axial plane:* parallel to the infraorbital meatal line, beginning at this line and ending on the supraorbital margin.

- *Coronal plane:* if possible at 90° to the axial scans. Scan from the anterior aspect of the globe to the anterior clinoid processes.

It is emphasised that all orbital scans should be performed with the eyes closed, in order to minimise eye movements.

Conditions

Thyroid eye disease – Axial and coronal scans, with 3 mm slice thickness and increment are used. No contrast enhancement is employed.

Retro-orbital lesions – Axial 3 mm scans through the orbit and 10 mm scans through the remainder of the brain are performed. This is repeated with contrast enhancement if any abnormality is detected.

Lacrimal gland tumours – Axial and coronal 3 mm scans before and after contrast enhancement are performed.

Periorbital infection – These also demand axial and coronal 3 mm scans before and after contrast enhancement. It may be necessary to scan a more extensive area to include the original source of infection, usually from the paranasal sinuses, using wider slice thicknesses and increments.

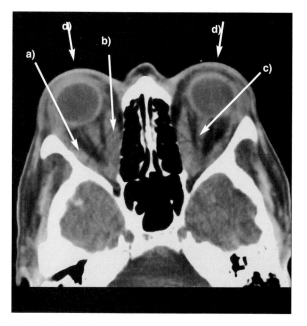

Figure 2.45 — Orbits. Axial projection in dysthyroid eye disease: a, thickened lateral rectus muscle; b, thickened medial rectus muscle; c, optic nerve; d, bilateral proptosis

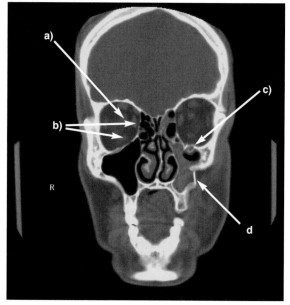

Figure 2.46 — Orbits and facial bones trauma. Coronal projection: a, optic nerve; b, ocular muscles; c, 'blow out' fracture of orbital floor showing 'tear drop' sign of herniation of orbital contents into antrum; d, fracture of left maxillary wall.

Angular dermoids – These lesions usually present in small children and are small swellings related to the inner or outer canthus of the eye. Slice thickness and increment of 1 mm are required to image the dermoid correctly, and the problems inherent in any paediatric scanning prevail. Often a short-acting general anaesthetic is given to ensure that a good quality scan is obtained. Axial scans with low exposure factors appropriate to the child's age should be performed. Contrast enhancement is rarely required.

Intraocular foreign bodies – CT is an excellent modality to assist in the localisation of intraocular foreign bodies particularly those which are non-metallic. A protocol is given in Table 2.18.

Petrous temporal bones

(Figures 2.47–2.49)

Indications for scans of this area include:

- cholesteatoma
- preselection assessment of cochleas in cochlear implant programme
- acoustic neuroma (see posterior fossa tumours, p. 21).

Scanning protocol for petrous temporal bones

This is given in Tables 2.19 and 2.20.

Table 2.18 – Protocol for visualising intraocular foreign bodies

PERFORM A SHORT AP SCAN PROJECTION RADIOGRAPH	
Patient position	Supine in head rest with radiographic baseline angled 15–20° craniocaudal.
Start position	Infraorbital margin
End position	Superior orbital margin
Gantry angle	Parallel to infraorbital meatal line
Protocol	
Slice thickness	1 mm
Table increment	1 mm
Kilovoltage	120 kV
mAs per slice	200 mAs
Algorithm	Detail
Scan field of view	25 cm
Display field of view	18 cm
Window width	300
Window level	20/40

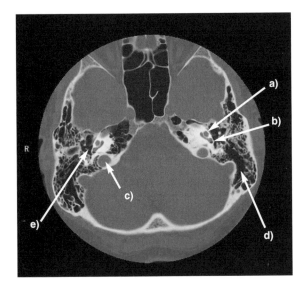

Figure 2.47 — Petrous temporal bones. A 1 mm axial section: a, apical turn of cochlea; b, basal turn of cochlea; c, jugular foramen; d, mastoid air cells; e, middle ear and ossicles.

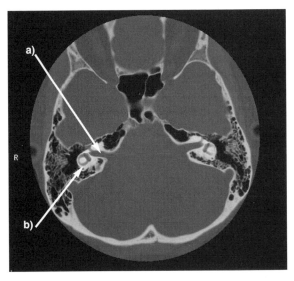

Figure 2.48 — Petrous temporal bones. A 1 mm axial section: a, internal auditory meatus; b, lateral semicircular canal

ADAPTATION FOR COCHLEAR IMPLANT ASSESSMENT

Patients may also have MRI to exclude acoustic neuroma. Axial scans are performed as above, but the number of scans should be limited to approximately 15 sections, from the lower third of the external auditory meatus to the internal auditory meatus, with a 15 cm display field of view.

Some centres also use direct coronal imaging for cochlear implant assessment. If it is difficult to obtain

Table 2.19 – Axial scan of petrous temporal bones:

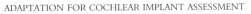

PERFORM LATERAL SCAN PROJECTION RADIOGRAPH

Patient position	Supine in head rest
Start position	Skull base
End position	Superior margin of petrous temporal bone
Gantry angle	30° cranial to infraorbital meatal line
Protocol	
Slice thickness	1 mm
Table increment	1 mm
Kilovoltage	140 kV
mAs per slice	300 mAs (150 mA: 2 sec scan-time)
Algorithm	Bone
Scan field of view	25 cm
Display field of view	18 cm
Window width	4000
Window level	750

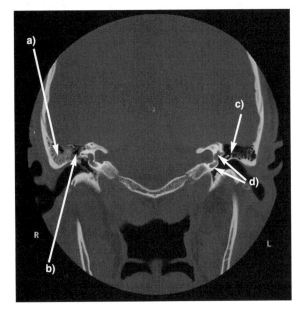

Figure 2.49 — Petrous temporal bones. A 1 mm coronal section: a, poorly aerated mastoid air cells; b, soft tissue cholesteatoma in attic of middle ear; c, normal ossicles; d, labyrinth of inner ear.

Table 2.20 – Coronal scan of petrous temporal bones:

PERFORM LATERAL SCAN PROJECTION RADIOGRAPH	
Patient position	Prone with head extended
Start position	Anterior margin of petrous temporal bone
End position	Posterior margin of petrous temporal bone
Gantry angle	90° to skull base of middle cranial fossa
Protocol	
Slice thickness	1 mm
Table increment	1 mm
Kilovoltage	140 kV
mAs per slice	300 mAs (150 mA: 2 sec)
Algorithm	Bone
Scan field of view	25 cm
Display field of view	18 cm
Window width	4000
Window level	750

coronal images directly. Good reformats can be made from the axial images but a more extensive series would have to be obtained.

Comments

Utilise fine focal spot by using a low mA of 150 and a 2 second scan time for all petrous temporal bone scanning. Do not use continuous (helical, spiral) scanning techniques for high definition bone work.

Stereotaxis

Scanning as part of stereotactic surgical or radiotherapy procedures is a large and complex subject and it is not within the scope of this chapter to describe this in any detail.

There are several different systems available, each requiring different mathematical localisation calculations and some of these involve computer analysis. Each operates on the principle of a base plate for the system, attached to the patients' head either by fixed skull pins or attached to an upper jaw mould. Various scanning, operating or treatment attachments can then be used on the fixed base plate, to precisely locate a biopsy probe or surgical instruments, or to focus radiotherapy beams.

The present writer's experience is with a Leksell frame which is attached to the outer table of the skull by pins

immediately prior to scanning and surgery and with the Gill–Thomas relocateable frame which is used for fractioned radiotherapy.

Most stereotactic frame types operate on a principle of fixed (vertical) and moveable (sloping) fiducial markers around the frame be it cylindrical (Gill–Thomas) or cuboid (Leksell). All types of frame are too large to be scanned using head size scan fields of view and therefore head algorithms are not available.

Each type of frame needs a specific table fixator. A typical protocol for stereotaxis is given in Table 2.21.

Table 2.21 – Typical protocol for stereotaxis

Slice thickness	1 mm
Table increment	1 mm
Kilovoltage	120 kV
mAs per slice	400 mAs
Algorithm	Standard
Scan field of view	35 cm
Display field of view	35 cm
Window width	250/100
Window level	40

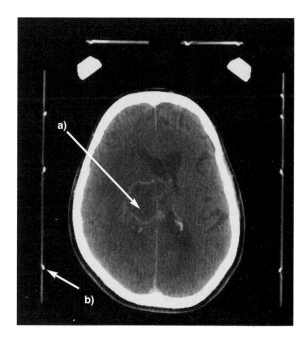

Figure 2.50 — Stereotaxis. Lexell stereotactic frame fixed for scan prior to biopsy: a, tumour to be biopsied; b, fiducial (10 in whole frame).

It is useful to magnify the image rather than to use a smaller display field of view to ensure inclusion of all fiducials.

Figures 2.50 shows a cerebral tumour being scanned prior to stereotactic biopsy using the Leksell frame and in Figure 2.51 the Gill–Thomas frame is being used to plan stereotactic therapy for a tumour.

Further reading

Banniser R (rev.) *Brain's clinical neurology.* Oxford Medical,

Dixon AK. *Body CT: a handbook.* Churchill Livingstone,

Draper IT. *Lecture notes on neurology.* Blackwell Scientific,

Ellis H, Logan B, Dixon A. *Human cross-sectional anatomy atlas of body sections and CT images.* Butterworth Heinemann,

McNaught AB. *Companion to illustrated physiology.* Churchill Livingstone.

McNaught AB, Callendar. *Illustrated physiology.* Churchill Livingstone.

Royal College of Radiologists. *Making the best use of a department of clinical radiology: guidelines for doctors.* London: Royal College of Radiologists,

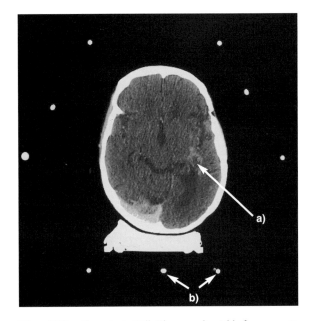

Figure 2.51 — Stereotaxis. Gill–Thomas relocatable frame scan to plan radiotherapy; a, tumour; b, fiducials (nine in total).

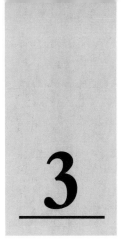

3

THE SPINE

Halina Szutowicz

Introduction

It is appropriate to say that the imaging modality of choice for the majority of spinal conditions is magnetic resonance (MR). However there will be many reasons why CT might still be used, not least for those patients who cannot tolerate the narrow 'tunnel' of most current designs of MR scanners, those who are just too large to fit into the MR scanner, or those who have implanted metal which means that MR scanning is contraindicated.

CT is essential when the requirement is for bone imaging of fractures in spinal trauma and for visualisation of foraminal stenosis, particularly in the cervical region.

There are situations where MR has failed to produce a definitive diagnosis or the MR findings do not correlate with the clinical observations and examination. This problem is particularly common in the cervical region and is resolved by the combination of cervical myelography plus CT and 3D reformatting to assess cervical root exit foramina.

In the writer's neurosurgical unit it is becoming the practice in spinal surgery to use some type of preoperative spinal marking under CT control to indicate accurately the correct level of interest and to thus minimise the surgery involved.

The lumbar spine

The two commonest reasons for imaging the lumbar spine are:

● Lumbar disc disease, most commonly at L5/S1 and L4/L5;

● Spinal stenosis, i.e. narrowing of either or both the spinal canal and lateral recesses.

Patient preparation and positioning

It is important to allow the patient with back pain to initially move onto the scanner couch in whatever way is most comfortable for them. Special care must be taken to assure the MRI-incompatible patient that the CT scanner has a wide aperture and is not tunnel-like. It may be appropriate to position the claustrophobic patient feet first into the scanner, although this may make cranial angulation of the gantry less tolerable to the patient, as most scanners have a wider 'funnel' to the rear of the gantry. The worried patients should also be reassured that the procedure is very quick and that

all that is required of them is to lie still for the duration of the scan.

All general lumbar spine scanning should be performed with the patient supine and the knees flexed over an appropriately angled wedge positioning pad or pillows. Arms should be lifted above the head and rested backwards onto a pillow. If the patient is unable to place the arms over the head then keeping the arms crossed high over the chest may be accepted.

Female patients of childbearing age should have their pregnancy risk established prior to the examination.

Use of 1 or 2 second scan times means breath-holding is not necessary.

It is beneficial to perform the lowest scans first. The maximum gantry angle will be used and the patient can be reassured that their knees will be moving away from the gantry. Always angle the gantry whilst standing beside the table, to reassure the patient; remote control when using large angles can be intimidating.

Lumbar disc disease

It is usually only necessary to examine the lowest three disc spaces and to perform a limited series at the L3/L4 level. Check the neurological findings against a nerve distribution chart if there is any doubt about the levels to be examined.

SCANNING PROTOCOL FOR LUMBAR DISC DISEASE
This is given in Table 3.1.

Table 3.1 – Protocol for lumbar disc disease

Scan projection radiographs	Both anteroposterior (AP) and lateral projections Length, 35 cm Zero to symphysis pubis, commence 35 cm superior 120–140 kV 40–160 mAs
Axial scans	
Slice thickness	3–5 mm
Table increment	3–5 mm
Algorithm	Standard
Kilovoltage	120–140 kV
mAs per slice	250–400 mAs
Scan field of view	48 cm
Display field of view	15 cm
Window width (WW)	500/1500
Window level (WL)	60/250

Measure the right or left, anterior or posterior offset positions from the scan projection radiographs and enter these into the axial scan protocol. Use the lateral scan projection radiograph (Figure 3.1) to plan the angles of the gantry and positions to scan, parallel to each disc space and covering the whole intervertebral foramen.

In the present writer's department, 5 mm sections overlapped by using a 4 mm table increment are routinely used; a 3 mm slice width and 3 mm increment can be used for very narrow disc spaces.

The L3/L4 disc space is examined using three 5 mm sections spaced 10mm apart, the middle section passing through the disc space, unless clinical symptoms relate to this level, in which case a full overlapping series should be performed with a limited series at L2/L3.

Comments

If the clinical information indicates disc lesions at a higher level than those most commonly scanned, these levels should be scanned in detail whilst restricting the other levels to a limited series. For example, unilateral sciatica will indicate a lateral disc lesion at L5/S1 or L4/L5, whereas bilateral sciatica could be caused by a central disc lesion at a higher level.

The scan projection radiographs can be imaged on a large format as a substitute for additional plain radiographs of the spine.

The imaging of the spine should be taken on both soft tissue and bone settings to distinguish between disc and bony compression of nerve roots.

Note – The posterior margin of lumbar intervertebral discs should appear either slightly concave or straight.

Figures 3.2 and 3.3 show sections through disc spaces in the lumbar spine.

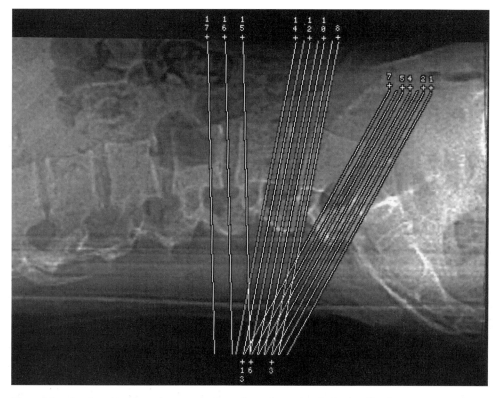

Figure 3.1 — Lumbar spine. Lateral scan projection radiograph; routine for lumbar disc disease.

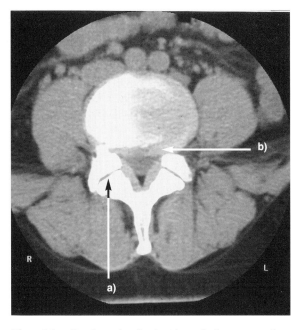

Figure 3.2 — Lumbar spine. Section through disc space: a, facet joint; b, disc protrusion.

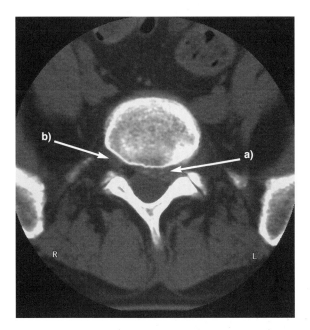

Figure 3.3 — Lumbar spine. A 5 mm section through L4/L5 disc space showing: a, disk prolapse to the *left* encroaching on exiting nerve root; b, normal exiting nerve root on *right*.

Spinal stenosis (Figure 3.4–3.6)

PROTOCOL FOR SPINAL STENOSIS

Perform anteroposterior and lateral scan projection radiographs as for disc disease. These patients are likely to be older and possibly larger than those with disc disease, so it may be necessary to use the higher values of the range of kilovoltage and mAs given for both scan projection radiographs and axial scans.

From the lateral scan projection radiograph, plan three axial sections through each disc space, from L5/S1 up to L1/L2, with the middle section passing through the middle of and parallel to each disc space. The axial scans should be 5 mm in thickness and separated using a table increment of 10 mm.

Lateral recess stenosis will be demonstrated on the lowest of each set of three sections and canal diameter assessed on the other two sections. If other pathology is demonstrated, then extra sections can be performed and intersected with the initial sequence.

Imaging should be on both soft tissue and bone settings, as in the section on disc disease.

Cervical spine

(Figures 3.7 and 3.8)

Foraminal stenosis

MR imaging should always be used to investigate cervical disc disease but, due to the lack of signal from bone, it is often very difficult to assess the degree of encroachment on cervical nerve roots from osteophyte formation within the intervertebral foramen. The 3D post processing of continuously acquired (helical) images can demonstrate the foramina accurately and allows for imaging of both external and internal surfaces of the vertebrae.

Patient preparation and positioning

The procedure is explained to the patient, and the need for keeping completely still is emphasised. Breath-holding is not necessary but very gentle breathing is required.

The patient's head is positioned in a radiolucent anatomical pad on the couch top, and the arms relaxed by the sides. If the lower cervical spine is to be imaged, traction straps can be used to keep the shoulders lowered and relaxed.

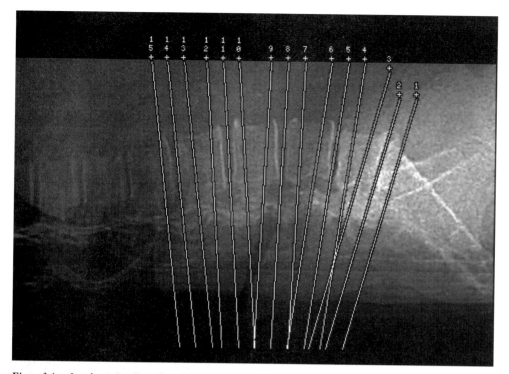

Figure 3.4 — Lumbar spine. Lateral scan projection radiograph: routine for spinal stenosis.

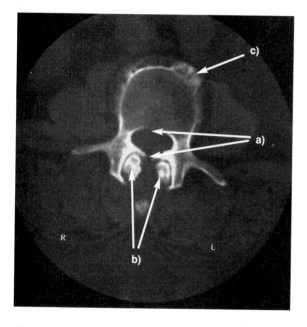

Figure 3.5 — Lumbar spine; spinal stenosis. A 5 mm axial section through upper lumbar vertebra showing: a, reduction of antero-posterior diameter of spinal canal (c.f. Figure 3.3); b, osteophytic changes in facet joints; c, anterior osteophyte on vertebral body.

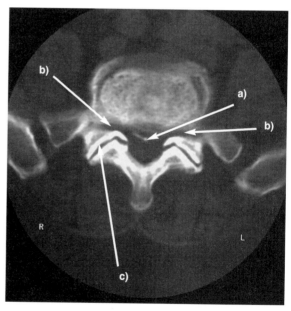

Figure 3.6 — Lumbar spine. A 5 mm axial section at L5/S1, disc level: a, central disc protrusion with some calcification within the disc; b, bilateral lateral recess stenosis from facet joint osteophytes; c, facet joint space.

The patient is aligned to axial, coronal and sagittal positioning lights to place the cervical spine in the centre of the scanning field.

Scanning protocol for the cervical spine

Details are given in Table 3.2.

The choice of axial scan thickness is dependent upon the area to be covered. A 3 mm thickness is usual if more than three vertebrae are to be studied. A gantry angle is selected which is appropriate to the angle of the disc spaces of the main area of interest.

Post scan processing is used to reconstruct 3 mm sections in 1 mm increments and to produce 3D images.

Table 3.2 – Scanning protocol for the cervical spine

Scan projection Radiograph	Lateral
	Length, 25 cm
	Zero to 5 cm above orbitomeatal baseline
	120 kV
	120 40–80 mA

Axial scans (helical)	
Slice thickness	1–3 mm
Table pitch	1–1.5
Algorithm	Standard
Kilovoltage	120 kV
mAs per slice	200–400 mAs
Scan field of view	25 cm
Display field of view	15 cm
Window width	500/1500
Window level	60/250

Lateral scan projection radiograph in major trauma (Figure 3.9)

It is frequently of value to perform a lateral scan projection radiograph of the cervical spine in patients having head CT for major head injury. It may have been difficult to obtain a conventional radiograph and shoulder traction may not be appropriate.

The flexibility of those scanners which allow a choice of exposure factors on scan projection radiographs enables a good image to be produced under most circumstances.

A protocol is given in Table 3.3.

Table 3.3 – Scanning protocol for cervical spine in major trauma

Lateral scan projection radiograph
Length, 30 cm
Zero to 5 cms above orbitomeatal baseline.
140 kV
40–200 mAs

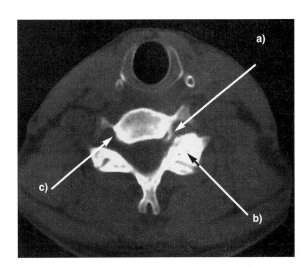

Figure 3.7 — Cervical spine. A 3 mm axial section showing: a, ostephyte compromising exit foramen on *left;* b, facet joint overgrowth on *left;* c, normal exit foramen on *right.*

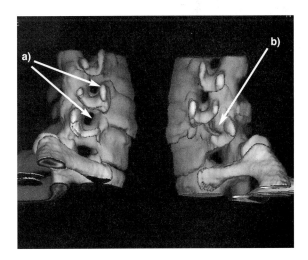

Figure 3.8 — Cervical spine. 3D reformat oblique views: a, normal intervertebral exit foramen; b, osteophyte formation obliterating intervertebral foramen.

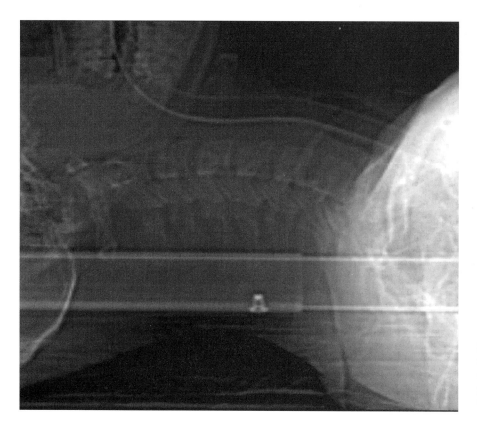

Figure 3.9 — Cervical spine. Lateral scan projection radiograph of trauma patient on spinal scoop: C_7–T_1 visualised.

Using the highest exposure settings if necessary, and varying the window widths and levels may produce reassuring information for clinicians.

Spinal trauma

The treatment and assessment of spinal fractures varies considerably from centre to centre. My experience is that the majority of spinal fractures do not require immediate imaging other than plain radiographs. CT is usually performed within 24–48 hours of the patient's admission to the spinal injury unit, when appropriate support is available, i.e. an orthopaedic spinal specialist or neurosurgeon and a neuroradiologist with interest in spinal trauma. It may also be necessary to have sufficient personnel available for safe patient transfer, according to the injury and the ward's patient movement protocol.

Rapid helical scanning has made the imaging of these problematic injuries much more efficient and 3D post processing is, in most cases, a valuable contribution to the full assessment of the injury. The extent of possible damage to the spinal cord is a clinical judgement and is assessed by neurological examination.

Some injuries to the cervical spine may need both CT and MR imaging in the acute stage to fully assess the damage to vital areas of the cervical spinal cord.

CT is required to fully visualise the bony injury and as such the examination can be conducted with lower exposure factors. CT examination will assess:

- the type of spinal fracture;
- whether the fracture is stable or unstable;
- the presence of fragments of bone within the spinal canal;
- facet joint disruption.

Axial scans can answer most of these questions but the ability to produce multiplanar reconstructions and 3D images, which can be viewed from any angle, is a vital component in the accurate assessment of the injury.

Scans of spinal injuries are shown in Figures 3.10–3.13.

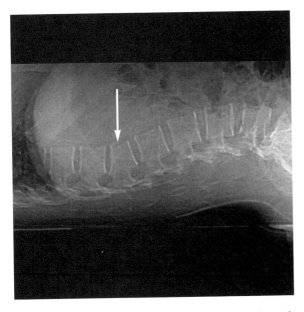

Figure 3.10 — Spinal trauma. Lateral scan projection radiograph showing fracture of body of L1

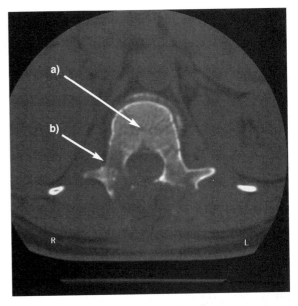

Figure 3.11 — Lumbar spine trauma. Axial section of same patient as Figure 3.10): a, fracture line through vertebral body; b, fracture through pedicle, not clearly visualised on lateral scan projection radiograph.

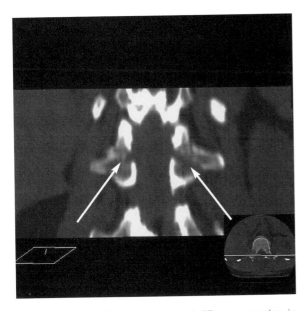

Figure 3.12 — Lumbar spine trauma. A 2D reconstruction in coronal plane showing extent of fractures (arrowed) through pedicles. The disrupted neural arch makes this an unstable spinal injury.

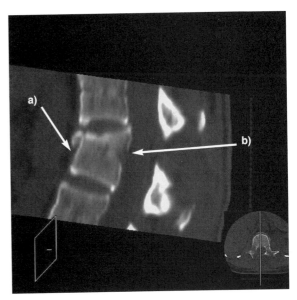

Figure 3.13 — Lumbar spine trauma. A 2D sagittal reconstruction: a, anterior wedging of vertebral body; b, posterior displacement and distraction of vertebral body.

Patient preparation and positioning

Good liasion with the spinal injury unit is essential. Spinal injury patients who have been in a specialist unit for 24 hours are well aware of their potential injury and have already become used to the care with which they are handled. Explanations to the patient can thus be restricted to information about the scan itself, the duration, table movements, noise, etc.

The patient is transferred to the scanner couch by whatever method is chosen by the spinal injuries team and every effort should be made to place the patient centrally on the couch.

Axial, coronal and sagittal positioning lights are used to centre the spine to the centre of the scanning field of view.

Scanning protocol for spinal injuries

The methods are the same whichever area of the spine is to be examined, and sensible judgement of exposure factors should be made on a case by case basis.

Table 3.4 – Scanning protocol for spinal injuries

Scan projection Radiographs	AP and lateral
	Length, 30–40 cm, for thoracic and lumbar spine; zeroed appropriately for the relevant area
	Length 25–30 cm for cervical spine; zero to 5 cm above orbitomeatal baseline
	120 kV
	40–100 mAs

AXIAL SCANS

Continuous volume acquisition (helical or spiral) scanning should be chosen for the axial images, using low mAs, as only bone detail is required. A standard algorithm should be used to acquire the data as this produces better 3D reconstructions. Relevant axial images may be post processed into bone algorithm. The axial acquisition should be performed with a gantry angulation appropriate to the area of the spine under examination.

It is vital to obtain good axial sections of the fracture site as well as good cover above and below. It is best to use a helical pitch of 1 whenever possible, to avoid image degradation, and the low mAs settings allow this, whilst keeping the radiation dose to a minimum.

Table 3.5 – Exposure protocols for spinal injuries

Thoracic and lumbar spine	
Slice thickness	5 mm
Table pitch	1 (up to 1.5)
Algorithm	Standard
Kilovoltage	120 kV
mAs per slice	160–320 mAs
Scan field of view	35–48 cm
Display field of view	18 cm
Window width	1000–1500
Window level	150–300
Post process	Into 3 mm increments

Cervical spine	
Slice thickness	3–5 mm
Table pitch	1–1.3
Algorithm	Standard
Kilovoltage	120 kV
mAs per slice	80–160 mAs
Scan field of view	25 cm
Display field of view	15 cm
Window width	1000–1500
Window level	150–250
Post process	Into 1 mm increments

Table 3.5 gives details of the exposure protocols for the thoracic lumbar and cervical spine.

CT myelography

Performance of CT myelography is extremely rare where there is an MR unit. However the factors mentioned previously, regarding patient size, claustrophobia, metallic implants and non-correlation of MR findings with patient symptomatology, may apply.

Following up myelography with CT imaging had become normal practice in the writer's unit, prior to the availability of MR scanning.

Cervical CT myelography

Following contrast introduction to the cervical region, either by direct lateral C1/C2 puncture or via a lumbar puncture and the use of table tilt, very narrow section CT axial images are needed to accurately demonstrate the cervical nerve root pockets.

Figures 3.14 and 3.15 are examples of CT myelography.

PATIENT PREPARATION AND POSITIONING

Following conventional myelography films, or simply the introduction of contrast medium, the patient remains supine with only one pillow. The scan can be performed up to 3 or 4 hours after the contrast introduction, provided the patient remains supine and relatively still. The patient is transferred to the CT couch and is positioned supine with the head in a radiolucent anatomical positioning pad. Axial, coronal and sagittal positioning lights are used to position the spine in the centre of the scanning field of view. The arms and shoulders can be given gentle traction with traction straps to enable better visualisation of the lower cervical vertebrae.

PROTOCOL FOR CERVICAL CT MYELOGRAPHY

Details are given in Table 3.6.

Table 3.6 – Scanning protocol for cervical CT myelography

Scan projection radiograph	Lateral
	Length, 25 cm
	Zero to 5 cm above orbitmeatal baseline.
	120 kV
	40–80 mAs
Axial scans (helical)	
Slice thickness	1–3 mm
Table pitch	1–1.5
Algorithm	Standard
Kilovoltage	120 kV
mAs per slice	200 mAs
Scan field of view	25 cm
Display field of view	15 cm
Window width	1000
Window level	150/200
Gentry angle	Parallel to main area of interest.

Note   In some large patients where imaging of the lower cervical region is required, it will be necessary to increase the size of the scan field of view and to increase the mAs value to accommodate scanning through the upper shoulders.

CT myelography of non-cervical spinal regions

Protocols are programmed to suit individual patient presentations. Following conventional myelographic imaging the area of pathology will have been identified by the total or partial block of cranial flow of contrast medium. CT is an essential adjunct to full diagnosis of the extent and possible nature of the lesion.

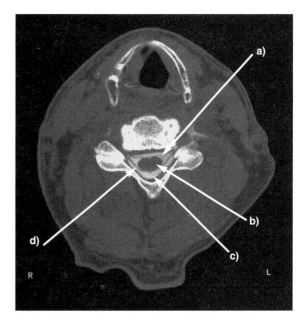

Figure 3.14 — CT myelography. Cervical spine: 1 mm axial section post-myelography: a, anterior nerve root; b, normal cervical spinal cord; c, contrast medium in spinal subarachnoid space; d, posterior nerve root.

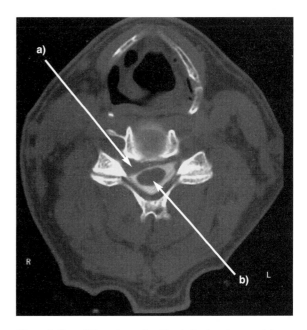

Figure 3.15 — CT myelography. Cervical spine: 1 mm axial section post-myelography. a, cervical disc protrusion compressing nerve root and compromising the exit foramen; b, distorted cervical spinal cord.

PATIENT PREPARATION AND POSITIONING

The patient is positioned supine on the CT couch, arms raised above the head and supported on pillows. The knees should be bent and supported with a wedge pad. Axial, coronal and sagittal positioning lights are used to centre the spine to the scan field of view. An explanation of the procedure is given and the need to keep completely still is emphasised.

AP and lateral scan projection radiographs are obtained to allow planning of the precise location of the axial sections. These views should demonstrate the contrast medium within the spinal subarachnoid space.

CT scans of the thoracic and lumbar spine are shown in Figures 3.16 and 3.17.

AXIAL SCANS

- If an apparently complete block to the cranial flow of contrast has been demonstrated 5 mm contiguous sections should be performed in a cranial direction, from the normal appearances below the block. It is usually possible to detect some contrast that has passed the block and thus determine the upper limit of the lesion when the normal spinal cord is again visualised.

- If the abnormality visualised on conventional myelography has demonstrated upper and lower limits, scans should be performed from above the lesion to below the lesion, thus demonstrating normal appearances of the cord as well as the abnormality. Axial sections of 5mm are usually appropriate, and a helical acquisition might also be appropriate on a pitch greater than 1 if the lesion is extensive.

PROTOCOL FOR NON-CERVICAL CT MYELOGRAPHY

Details are given in Table 3.7.

Biopsy and preoperative spinal marking

Patients for biopsy or spinal marking will already have had CT or MR examinations. However it will be necessary to relocate the lesion or level for marking, using a vertical gantry for accuracy of needle positioning.

Patient preparation and positioning

The procedure is explained to the patient prior to positioning on the CT couch, and a consent form should be signed.

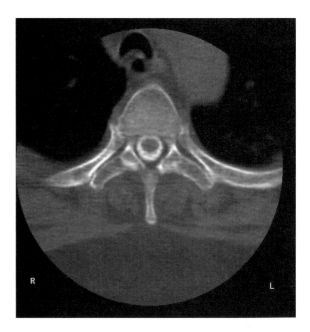

Figure 3.16 — CT myelography. Thoracic spine: contrast in spinal subarachnoid space; normal appearances.

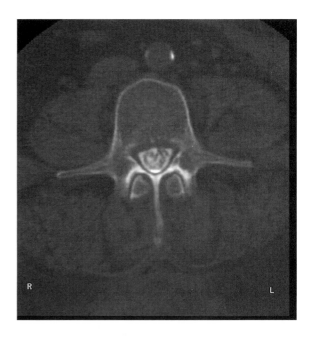

Figure 3.17 — CT myelography. Lumbar spine: contrast in spinal subarachnoid space surrounding the lumbar nerve roots of the cauda equina; normal appearances.

Table 3.7 – Scanning protocol for non-cervical CT myelography

Scan projection radiographs	AP and lateral Length, 30–40 cm Zero appropriately for the area under examination 120 kV 40–160 mAs
Axial scans (contiguous)	
Slice thickness	5 mm
Table increment	5 mm
Algorithm	Standard
Kilovoltage	120 kV
mAs per slice	200 mAs
Scan field of view	48 cm
Display field of view	18 cm
Window width	1000
Window level	150/200
Axial scans (helical)	
Slice thickness	5 mm
Pitch	1–1.5
Algorithm	Standard
Kilovoltage	120 kV
mAs per slice	200 mAs
Scan field of view	48 cm
Display field of view	18 cm
Window width	1000
Window level	150/200
Gantry angle	Selected as appropriate for area under examination

It should be emphasised that keeping perfectly still is of vital importance. Breath-holding may be required if the procedure is to be in the thoracic region.

The patient is positioned prone on the CT couch with the arms raised above the head and resting on a pillow; the head can be turned to one side. The lower legs are supported on a pillow.

Axial, coronal and sagittal positioning lights are used to centre the spine to the centre of the scan field of view.

Scanning protocol for biopsy or spinal marking

Details are given in Table 3.8.

The use of a 25 cm display field of view will visualise the skin surface on the optimal section.

To check needle positions, a much lower exposure technique may be utilised, e.g. 150 mAs and a lower

detail matrix may speed up image processing time on some systems. Utilise the biopsy protocols on scanner systems to produce an odd number of narrow (3 mm) sections centred on the marker or biopsy needle entry point. Short length helical scan technique can also be a valuable tool in biopsy scanning.

Table 3.8 – Protocol for biopsy or spinal marking

Scan projection radiographs	Posteroanterior and lateral Length, 30–40 cm Zero appropriately for the area under examination 120 kV 40–80 mAs
Axial scans (contiguous)	
Slice thickness	3 mm
Table increment	3 mm
Algorithm	Standard
Kilovoltage	120 kV
mAs per slice	300 mAs
Scan field of view	48 cm
Display field of view	25 cm
Window width	500/1500
Window level	60/250

Spinal marking (Figure 3.18)

Methylene blue is introduced via a vertical spinal needle into the ligamentum flavum at the level of the operative lumbar disc lesion and on the side of maximum disc prolapse. The blue dye can also be left in the needle track to guide a minimally invasive surgical approach. This procedure must be done within 24 hours prior to surgery.

It is also possible to use hook needles to mark levels in the thoracic spine.

Spinal biopsy (Figure 3.19)

Bone and/or soft tissue biopsies of spinal and paraspinal lesions will normally be taken using a posterolateral approach. Localisation of the optimal slice position is performed as for spinal marking above. The measurements of angle and depth of approach are made from the skin surface on the image.

Confirmation of position is made using the same technique as described above for spinal marking.

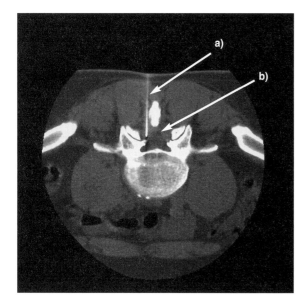

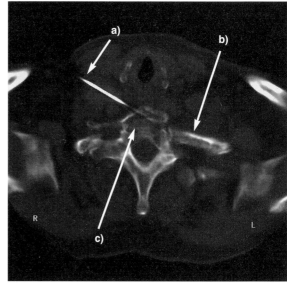

Figure 3.18 — Preoperative spinal marking. Lumbar spine: a, needle in position in ligamentum flavum; b, ligamentum flavum.

Figure 3.19 — Spinal biopsy. Biopsy of T1 vertebral body a) bone biopsy needle; b, first rib; c, abnormal vertebral body. (N.B. supine patient position)

Further reading

Bannister R (rev.) *Brain's clinical neurology.* Oxford Medical,

Dixon AK. *Body CT: a handbook.* Churchill Livingstone,

Draper IT. *Lecture notes on neurology.* Blackwell Scientific,

Ellis H, Logan B, Dixon A. *Human cross-sectional anatomy atlas of body sections and CT images.* Butterworth Heinemann,

McNaught AB. *Companion to illustrated physiology.* Churchill Livingstone,

McNaught AB, Callendar. *Illustrated physiology.* Churchill Livingstone,

Royal College of Radiologists. *Making the best use of a department of clinical radiology: guidelines for doctors.* London: Royal College of Radiologists,

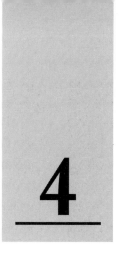

4

THE THORAX

Shelagh Smith

Introduction

Cross-sectional imaging of the thorax using computed tomography provides a simple, non-invasive demonstration of all structures of the thorax. It can often identify confusing superimposed shadows seen on the plain film chest radiograph.[1] It is recognised primarily as an accepted technique to provide diagnosis, differentiation and staging of the course of pulmonary or mediastinal disease.[2]

CT imaging techniques and identification of attenuation values may determine diagnosis, while CT guidance is widely used for intervention – biopsy, aspiration or drainage. In the staging of malignant disease CT provides important information for the surgeon and oncologist,[3] and CT is routinely used in the planning of radiotherapy treatment.

General note – CT scanning of the thorax is not usually performed in isolation. Other investigations and/or imaging modalities may be required to complement or supplement the information obtained. Other areas may need to be scanned, to look for source or spread of disease[3] or extent of trauma. Protocols for such scanning are discussed elsewhere.

Helical versus conventional CT

The advent of helical CT scanning has greatly increased the potential of CT imaging of the thorax. Short acquisition times, utilising a combination of slip-ring technology, patient translation, movement reduction algorithms, higher powered X-ray tubes with rapid heat dissipation and more efficient X-ray detectors, allow the entire thorax to be imaged in a matter of seconds. Most importantly this usually means within a single breath-hold.[4]

CT imaging of the thorax may necessitate demonstration of the bony thoracic cage and the soft tissue structures within, in their entirety, or it may focus on a particular organ or pathology. One or all of the following areas may be included:

- pleural cavity
- mediastinum
- cardiovascular structures
- bony cage of ribs and sternum

All of these structures move on respiration, therefore single breath-hold scanning techniques have revolutionised CT thorax scanning. This and other advantages of helical scanning of the thorax are listed below.

Advantages of thoracic helical CT scanning

- The data is continuous, because a whole volume is scanned.[5]

- Small areas of pathology are unlikely to be missed; this can happen with conventional CT scanning if the slices are not contiguous.[5]

- The whole volume can be scanned in one breath-hold, so there is no misregistration of data due to respiratory movement.[4]

- Contrast enhancement is more uniform throughout the study so the amount used may be reduced, optimised and captured to perform CT angiography, or multiphased studies.[5]

- It can be faster for the patient; this has excellent indications for paediatric, geriatric and trauma scanning, and for increasing workloads.[5]

- Image manipulation, such as multiplanar (MP) and three-dimensional (3D) reformatting of images, shaded surface displays (SSDs) and maximum intensity projections (MIPs), has expanded and improved because the continuous data acquisition allows overlapping slices and reconstruction at any point within the volume of raw data.[5] This has helped to make CT angiography a reality.

- Advanced 3D postprocessing techniques are now being developed to allow a simulated view from inside a lumen or anatomical space, indicating that intraluminal angiography and simulated bronchoscopy may be examinations of the future.[6]

- A radiation dose reduction is indicated because the likelihood of repeat scans due to patient movement is reduced. Also the scans are undertaken at a lower mAs value because of the high tube output required for spiral CT scanning: this is a direct reduction of radiation dose.[7]

It can be seen that the benefits to the patient and imaging department of fast volume data acquisition are manifold. There are of course some disadvantages which are generally outweighed by the advantages, and which are reducing with rapidly improving CT technology. They do, however, warrant a mention.

Disadvantages of thoracic helical CT scanning

- Helical CT scanning requires an X-ray tube capable of constant high tube loadings.[5]

- For high resolution scanning at very thin slice thickness, the spatial resolution may be reduced.[5]

- The special helical reconstruction algorithm may take longer to reproduce the image.[5]

- There is a tendency to over-reconstruct data; a reconstruction interval of approximately 2 per slice thickness provides adequate data for image manipulation.[8]

Observational disadvantages:

- Advanced image manipulation techniques are at the moment quite slow, and operator-dependent, and the simulated image may not provide truly accurate diagnostic information.

Use of conventional CT

In practice helical scanning for the thorax has now become routine for CT imaging, and in the main is used for diagnostic purposes. There are a few instances where conventional CT may still be preferred and these are listed below.

- High resolution (HR) CT for detailed imaging of lung parenchyma, differentiation of pulmonary nodules and focal lung disease. Incremental acquisition using narrow beam collimation, in the writers' experience, is still the protocol of choice. Nevertheless, studies are beginning to show that helical acquisition may provide similar information, since a volume acquisition allows data to be reconstructed retrospectively (Figure 4.1), to overlap slices directly through the centre of pulmonary nodules[9,10] or areas of interest. This provides more information without further scanning of the patient and reduces partial volume artefact: however the detail may not be equal to that of incremental scanning.

- Biopsy, aspiration, drainage. Although helical acquisition is useful for identification of a lesion or collection, it has little advantage over conventional scanning for accurate localisation. It has previously been suggested that the interpolation algorithms employed for image reconstruction, may produce a less than accurate representation. In practice, however, it seems to make little difference.

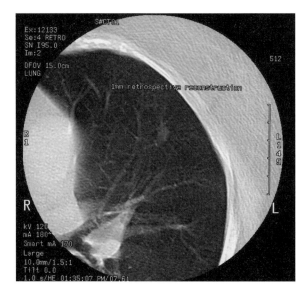

Figure 4.1 — A 1 mm retrospective reconstruction of a routine unenhanced scan on a lung algorithm, for differentiation of a small area of shadowing in the left anterior upper lobe.

- Radiotherapy planning. Helical CT is not widely used as yet because patient translation along the z-axis and image interpolation may affect treatment planning. 3D reformatting, though, can be used to aid planning.[11]

If a helical acquisition is not an option then conventional slice by slice scanning using contiguous slices clustered together, if possible, to reduce the number of breath-holds, will provide information similar to that of helical scanning.

Techniques and protocols in this chapter

For the purposes of this chapter, the scanning techniques and parameters refer to a helical acquisition unless otherwise stated, since from experience it appears that helical scanning of the thorax provides the optimal examination for all concerned. Indeed, if the present sales literature is to be believed, all scanners on the market now have a helical option indicating that it will become more widely available.

The techniques and protocols described here have been performed using either the ProSpeed or HiSpeed Advantage CT scanners in conjunction with the Advantage Windows workstation, all from GE Medical Systems, (Milwaukee, Wisconsin, USA). The techniques and protocols stated, therefore, refer to the software and hardware available on these scanners. The terminology used also relates to these scanners since there is no universal CT terminology.

The techniques and protocols described in the following text are in regular use in the writers' CT scanning department. They have evolved from experience and are in no way static. They are effective at this time, but as knowledge increases with experience they are constantly being updated. In addition they are not advocated as the only correct methods but as those that work for the department in question, given the type and amount of CT thorax requests that are dealt with.

The CT thorax request

There is no doubt that a CT scan of the thorax can provide the clinician with a wealth of information and it is regarded as the examination of choice for any patient with abnormal or equivocal findings on a chest X-ray,[12] but if the findings are insignificant with respect to the patient's management then its necessity is in doubt. CT scanning is responsible for at least 20–30% of all medical radiation exposures[13] and, compared to a plain film chest radiograph, it uses a relatively high dose of ionising radiation. It is therefore extremely important that strict guidelines are adhered to when CT scans are requested, preferably with some input from a radiologist. For example, a CT scan of the thorax will demonstrate a pleural effusion[1] (Figure 4.2), but so will a chest X-ray. If the clinical question is the type and underlying cause of a pleural effusion then a CT scan may be

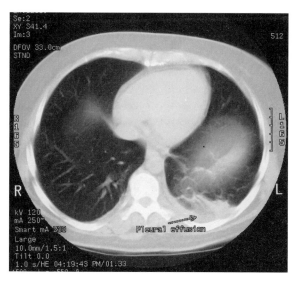

Figure 4.2 — Pleural effusion in the base of the left lung.

indicated, but clinical techniques and chest X-rays should be used to monitor its progression.

Once the necessity for a CT thorax scan has been confirmed, the scan should be performed in such a way as to keep the dose to the patient as low as diagnostically possible. An effective way of doing this is to have an efficient set of protocols in place which identify a standard or routine thorax protocol which may be tailored or supplemented to suit the patient's symptoms and answer the clinical question. The following scanning techniques and parameters aim to do this.

Routine unenhanced technique and parameters for thoracic CT

Preparation

This may begin as early as when the patient makes the appointment or is on the ward as an inpatient: for the patient to have prior information about the in-patient procedure that has been requested is good background preparation. Information leaflets at reception, in the waiting room or sent to the ward are useful. Any allergy or asthma history should be obtained as early as possible if steroid cover is to be arranged for intravenous (IV) contrast administration, dependent upon departmental policy.

The scanning procedure should be explained clearly and concisely to the patient as well as the necessity and purpose of oral and IV contrast. The patient should be given an idea as to the duration of the examination and told how they can communicate with the radiographer. Reassurance that they can be heard and spoken to often helps patients, as well as a frequent update as to how well the procedure is progressing. In the writer's experience, an explanation as to why it may appear to the patient that, on occasion, nothing is happening, is useful; this is when patients may become anxious and is often due to the radiographers' concentration on the images rather than on the patient! This may be the 10th scan of the day, but to the patient it is the one and only and can make a lasting impression; a relaxed patient is a still one making the procedure easier for everyone.

Breath-holding techniques are very important for thorax scanning and should, therefore, be explained to, and practised with the patient.

All patient details, as far as possible, should be entered prior to positioning the patient since this also reduces the time the patient is lying in the scanner.

The patient should be wearing a radiolucent gown and jewellery should have been removed from the area to be examined.

Positioning

This is extremely important: time spent making the patient comfortable will result in a high quality scan because the patient is more likely to keep still. Although the actual scanning time is short, the length of time the patient is on the scan table often seems long since the planning and checking of scans can be time consuming.

- The patient is positioned supine and usually head first into the gantry. Patients are often breathless, making it difficult for them to lie flat and so they may need to be propped up on pillows. This can make it difficult to feed the patient into the gantry so, if the scanner has a long enough table scan range to allow this, or with careful positioning, the patient can be positioned feet first. This is also more tolerable to the claustrophobic patient since their head does not have to go through the gantry. A pillow under the knees can also make the patient more comfortable. For a restless or nervous patient immobilisation straps may make them feel more secure.

- Centre, using laser centring lights, to the sternal notch, in the midline and in the mid-axillary line.

- Both arms should be raised above the head. This is sometimes not possible and may result in streak artefact across the images. To avoid or reduce this the following options or a combination of them may compensate:

- raise one arm if possible;

- increase exposure;

- change the algorithm to soft rather than standard to reduce noise on the image.

Scout view

This is the planning scan and is usually an anteroposterior (AP) view with the tube at 0° (Figure 4.3) An additional lateral scout view at 90° (Figure 4.4) may or may not be useful. The scout range usually covers a distance 250 – 350cms, depending upon the size of the patient to include from above the sternal notch to below the diaphragms, and is often programmed into the scan protocol. It is a relatively low dose scan compared to the main scans, generally using 120kVp, and 60–100mAs.[8]

Scan parameters

- The scan is planned from above the apices to below the diaphragms, centred in the midline and mid-axillary line.

- A slice thickness of 10 mm is adequate although 7 or 8 mm may be preferable if the scanner allows.[8]

- A 10 mm reconstruction interval is usually adequate, although with a helical acquisition a smaller reconstruction interval is possible if required.[8]

- Suspended respiration is important for thorax imaging. Practising with the patient and hyperventilation

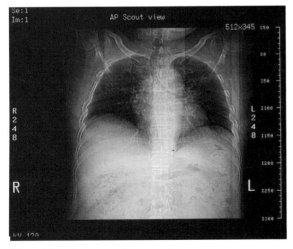

Figure 4.3 — Anteroposterior scout view.

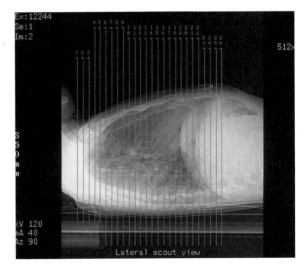

Figure 4.4 — Lateral scout view with scan reference lines.

immediately prior to scanning, may enable a longer breath-hold. For a very breathless patient it may be advisable to scan from the diaphragms up: the apices move less than the diaphragms on respiration, so limiting movement artefact. If breath-holding is impossible, gentle breathing may be better since the movement reduction algorithm of helical scanning may remove some artefact. In practice, scans performed in this manner are usually of a reasonable diagnostic quality.

- A helical acquisition using a pitch of 1.5 provides the ability to complete the scan in a single breath-hold as well as reducing the exposure to the patient.[8] However, it will also slightly increase the effective slice thickness and has the potential of reducing the definition, due to the increased speed of movement along the z-axis.[11] In practice, the benefits of a single breath-hold scan outweigh any loss of definition and the diagnostic value does not appear to be significantly reduced.

- A standard algorithm is the preferred algorithm for soft tissue imaging of the thorax. A soft algorithm may be selected instead of standard to aid noise reduction from streak artefacts caused by any dense objects, such as arms, valve replacement, pacemaker, or if the patient is larger than average. Both the standard and soft tissue algorithm provide good low-contrast resolution for demonstrating the soft tissue structures within the thorax (Figure 4.5) allowing structures of similar densities to be clearly delineated.[5]

- A lung, detail or bone algorithm should be used to reconstruct the raw data, in addition to the standard or soft algorithm and imaged using settings to demonstrate the lung parenchyma. Figure 4.6, when compared with Figure 4.7, demonstrates the difference in detail obtained by selecting different algorithms, although similar settings were used for imaging.

- The bony thoracic cage may be demonstrated by reconstructing the raw data on a bone algorithm and imaged using the appropriate bone settings (Figure 4.8). The lung, detail or bone algorithms utilise a 'high pass' filter which filters out the lower frequencies providing an image with high contrast resolution.[5]

- A 512 matrix is used.[8]

- Scan field of view (FOV): approximately 48 cms[8] but may be altered to suit patient size.

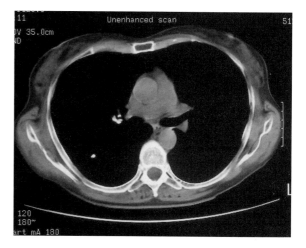

Figure 4.5 — Thorax scan reconstructed using a standard algorithm and imaged on mediastinum settings.

- Display FOV: approximately 35 cm[8] depending on patient size.

- Exposure factors are relatively low compared to CT scanning of other areas due to the presence of air in the lungs. Routinely used exposure factors are 120 kVp, and 100–200mA.[8] If only the lung parenchyma is to be demonstrated the exposure can be kept to the lower limit.

Viewing and Imaging

The resulting images can be viewed and reported from the scan monitor allowing manipulation of the images to the best advantage. However, this is not usually practicable since the radiologist will need time to review the images and this can hold up scanning. A remote workstation is an ideal solution, providing the radiologist with image manipulation facilities similar to those of scanning software. A report could then be provided without the need of a hard copy, but in reality, the demands of the clinician or surgeon, or the lack of available workstation means that a hard copy is required.

In the writer's opinion, if the radiologist reports from a workstation, and provided all the generated images are archived, the hard copy need only be a token documentation of the relevant images of the study.

The images should be viewed or imaged according to the tissue type under examination. This is done by 'windowing'[5] (See the CT terminology section at the beginning of the book). Suggested window widths and

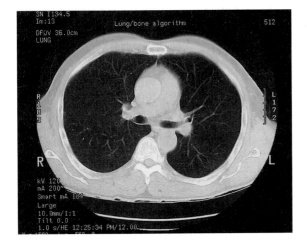

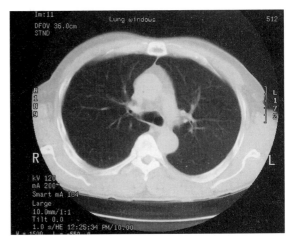

Figure 4.6 — Thorax scan reconstructed using a lung algorithm and imaged using lung settings The lung parenchyma is clearly delineated.

Figure 4.7 — Thorax scan reconstructed on a standard algorithm and imaged on lung settings. This does not delineate lung parenchyma with as much resolution as a lung algorithm.

levels used to provide optimum visualisation of structures of the thorax are as follows:

- mediastinum/soft tissue structures: 350 WW, 40 WL
- Lung parenchyma: 1500 WW, -550 WL
- Bone: 2500 WW, 250 WL

The difference in information obtained by windowing for the appropriate tissue can be seen in Figures 4.5 and 4.7.

The images printed onto hard copy should include the scout view(s) with and without scan reference lines (Figures 4.3 and 4.4).

Region of interest (ROI) measurements can be made on any abnormal area which will provide an attenuation measurement to indicate the type of tissue demonstrated and may offer a non-invasive definitive diagnosis.[14]

Figure 4.9 demonstrates a substance in the pleural cavity with CT numbers between 11 and 21; a fluid more dense than water which has a CT number of 0. This patient was found to have a haemothorax.

Comparison of ROIs pre and post contrast enhancement, can be useful to demonstrate any difference in tissue enhancement. ROI measurements should be documented along with the images. Multiplanar (MP), 3D reformatted images and shaded surface display (SSD) images may be produced from overlapping reconstructed slices to demonstrate the lungs and airways from viewpoints different from the axial scans.

These can be time consuming, and operator-dependent, and are only worthwhile if they significantly contribute to the patient's management.

The above description is of a routinely used protocol for CT scanning of the thorax. It can be used to demonstrate the organs of the thoracic cavity, unenhanced imaging of the mediastinum, the bony cage of the

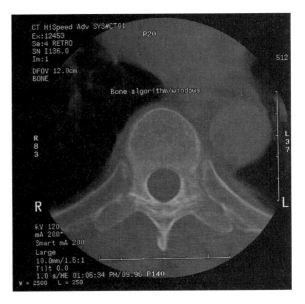

Figure 4.8 — A retrospective reconstruction through a thoracic vertebra, using a bone algorithm and imaged on bone settings, provides the best bone detail.

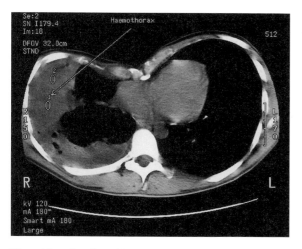

Figure 4.9 — A region of interest (ROI) measurement of the area under examination can assist in determining the type of effusion present: a mean CT number of 21, as demonstrated, suggests a fluid denser than water. This this was diagnosed as a haemothorax.

thorax and any associated pathology. CT visualisations of these structures are shown in Figures 4.10–4.19, demonstrating normal appearances, incidental findings and anomalies and abnormalities.

Contrast media

The correct and timely administration of contrast media can increase the amount of information gained from the unenhanced thorax scan. A contrast-enhanced

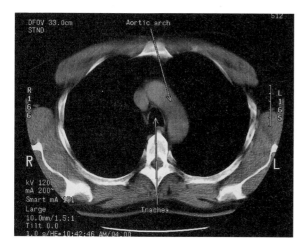

Figure 4.10. — Unenhanced routine thorax scan at the level of the aortic arch.

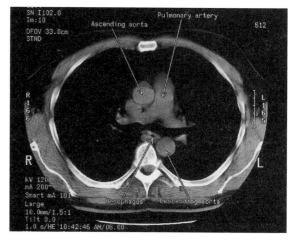

Figure 4.11 — Unenhanced routine thorax scan at the level of the main pulmonary artery.

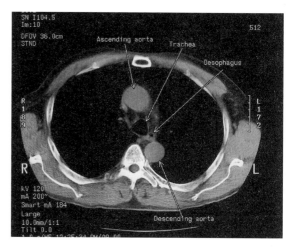

Figure 4.12 — Unenhanced routine thorax scan demonstrating the main structures of the mediastinum.

scan alone may be all that is indicated or it may be used in addition to the unenhanced scan. Intravenous administration of a contrast medium is the route most commonly used in CT scanning of the thorax, although an oral contrast medium may be used for demonstration of the oesophagus.

Oral contrast medium

Experience has shown that this is not commonly used in thorax scanning since its passage through the oesophagus is often too rapid to be captured on the scan. The main use, however, would be to outline the oesophagus and so

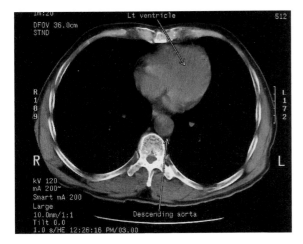

Figure 4.13 — Unenhanced routine thorax scan.

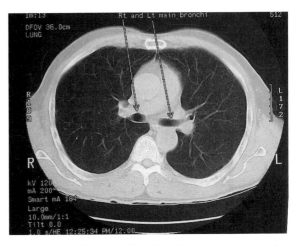

Figure 4.14 — Unenhanced routine thorax scan demonstrating lung parenchyma and main bronchi.

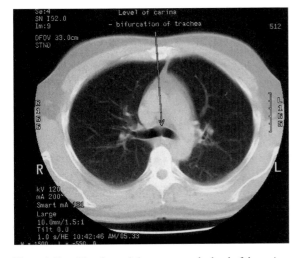

Figure 4.15 — Unenhanced thorax scan at the level of the carina.

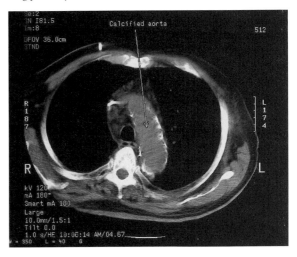

Figure 4.16 — Incidental finding on routine unenhanced scan, demonstrating a calcified aortic arch.

demonstrate any irregularity or pathology. Comparison of Figure 4.12 with Figure 4.20 demonstrates differences between the oesophagus scanned with and without oral contrast; the amount of extra information gained is debatable, but it may be useful. Routinely, however, a barium swallow would be the examination of choice for diagnosis, using CT scanning for staging and identifying spread of the disease.[3]

USING ORAL CONTRAST TO DEMONSTRATE THE OESOPHAGUS: PROTOCOL

An oral, water-soluble contrast medium such as Iopamidol; 10 ml to 150 ml of water, is suggested.

The barium sulphate type of CT oral contrast medium can be used, as its viscosity will allow it to travel more slowly through the oesophagus, but its density may cause streak artefacts and so detract from the images. Also the contraindications should be noted prior to administration.

The patient should be positioned as for a routine thorax scan. The scout view, as well as an unenhanced scan if necessary, is completed.

The patient should then be asked to drink approximately 100–150 ml of oral contrast. This is most easily done using a flexible straw, but it must be remembered that it is very difficult to drink when lying flat.

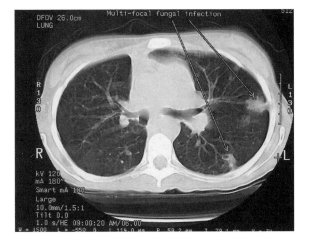

Figure 4.17 — Multi-focal fungal infection demonstrated on routine unenhanced thorax scan.

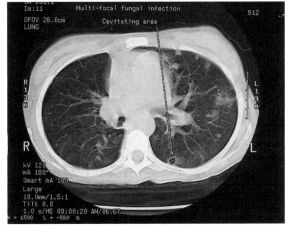

Figure 4.18 — Cavitation caused by fungal infection.

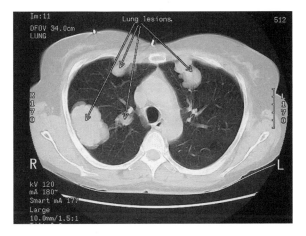

Figure 4.19 — Multiple lesions demonstrated on a routine unenhanced thorax scan; shown histologically to be pulmonary metastases.

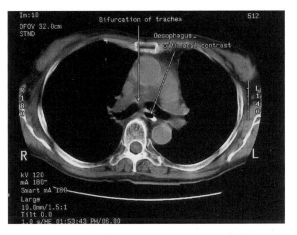

Figure 4.20 — Oesophagus outlined by an oral contrast medium.

Other scan parameters are as for routine mediastinum imaging, reducing the FOV and centring over the area of interest as appropriate. The scan should then start immediately the patient has finished drinking or, if possible, ask the patient to hold some of the fluid in their mouth until instructed to swallow. Again this can be quite difficult and often impractical, another reason why this procedure is not the examination of choice.

Intravenous contrast media

This is used routinely in thoracic scanning in order to demonstrate the vasculature of the mediastinum and pleural cavity, and is particularly useful where there is confusion between lymph nodes and vessels; Figures 4.21 and 4.22 demonstrate the difference between unenhanced and enhanced scans.

The fast scanning times of a helical acquisition allow optimisation of contrast media which, together with an appropriate time delay after administration and scanning with a single breath-hold, can demonstrate an organ in its entirety or in a particular vascular phase. This technique has made possible new techniques using non-invasive CT angiography, although the latter still requires more study and better understanding of interpretation before it can be widely accepted as a replacement for conventional methods of angiography.[15]

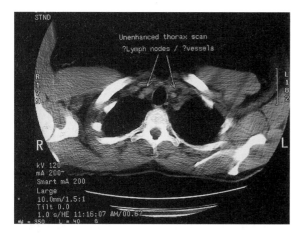

Figure 4.21. — Unenhanced thorax scan Differentiation between lymph nodes and vessels is questionable.

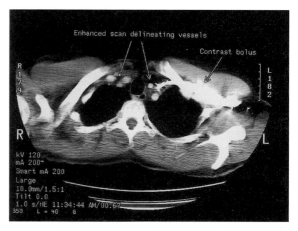

Figure 4.22. — Administration of an intravenous (IV) contrast medium clearly differentiates between lymph nodes and vessels.

A non-ionic contrast medium is preferred. Although it is more costly, it is safer for the patient and optimisation with helical techniques allows smaller volumes to be used.[6] The way in which the medium is administered depends largely upon the clinical question. This can range from a general investigation of the organ, vascular and nodal involvement in the staging of malignant disease,[3] or more specifically the query may concern the presence of an acute central pulmonary embolus[16] or thoracic aortic aneurysm.[17]

The type of contrast medium, its administration, the scanning delays and what may be demonstrated by its use will be identified in the following suggested protocols.

Suggested protocols

These are all based on the routine thorax protocol already described, supplemented or tailored to demonstrate or rule out a particular pathology and to answer the clinical question.

One of the benefits of CT scanning is that although it should only be requested in order to answer a specific clinical question, the amount of information obtained from one scan may do more than this: for instance it may allow diagnosis and staging of a disease in one examination. However, because of the high doses of radiation involved CT should not be considered as a screening test. A disadvantage to CT is that it may highlight an asymptomatic condition, posing the problem of treatment or leaving well alone.

Demonstration of the pleural cavity and mediastinum

This is indicated for:

- Diagnosis of malignant disease in the pleura, bronchi or mediastinum: to demonstrate any tumour and its extent.[2]

- Staging of malignant disease: to indicate whether it is operable; involvement with other organs, vasculature and lymph nodes; progression of disease pre and post treatment.[3,18]

- Diagnosis of pulmonary metastases.[2]

- Staging of metastatic disease: the number and size of pulmonary metastases can indicate the stage of a malignant disease.[3]

- Lymphadenopathy.[3]

- Lung and airway disease.[6]

- Pulmonary collapse.[19]

- Thymoma: myasthenia gravis may be due to a thymoma and it is, therefore, important for the patient's management to determine whether it is malignant.[20]

- Trauma: prior to helical CT this was not necessarily an indication; however where there are severe chest injuries it can rapidly provide the clinician with an overview of the patient's condition.

- Lung transplant assessment.[6,17]

Protocol for pleural cavity/mediastinum

A routine unenhanced CT thorax scan as previously described, may be performed, in the case of trauma accepting the patient's position as much as possible. This may be adequate alone but contrast enhancement will greatly increase the amount of information obtained.

An enhanced scan should be performed if vascular or nodal involvement is in question, and both pre and post contrast scans should be performed routinely for comparison in initial staging scans. From then on, either one alone may be indicated depending on the departmental protocol.

It is usually only necessary to have one set of reconstructions on a lung algorithm and lung settings, either pre or post contrast enhancement.

In the case of trauma where time is important, a single enhanced scan will give maximum information.

Enhanced scan parameters are similar to those of the routine unenhanced scan, following the administration of 50 – 100 ml of an intravenous, preferably non-ionic, contrast medium, 350 mg iodine/ml. This is usually administered through the ante-cubital vein at a rate of 2 ml/s., either by hand or pump injection.

The scan should be initiated after 30 sec. allowing optimal visualisation of the mediastinal vessels. Scans performed in this way can be seen in Figures 4.23–4.25 and comparisons can be made with the unenhanced images.

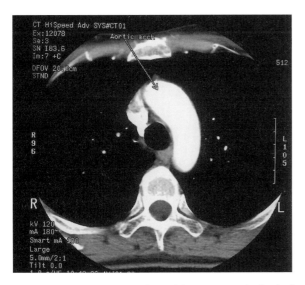

Figure 4.23. — IV contrast-enhanced thorax scan at the level of the aortic arch. Comparison can be made with Figure 4.10.

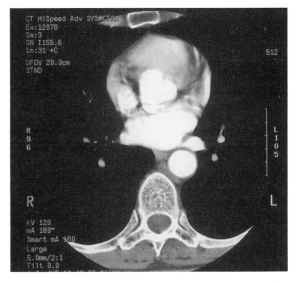

Figure 4.24. — IV contrast-enhanced scan demonstrating cardiovascular vessels. Comparison can be made with unenhanced images.

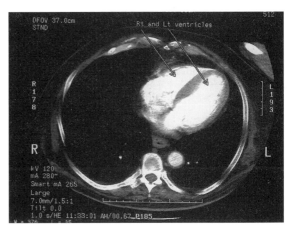

Figure 4.25. — IV contrast enhanced thorax scan demonstrating left and right ventricles and septum. Comparison can be made with Figure 4.13.

These scans should be imaged using settings similar to those used for the unenhanced scan.

CT angiography of the mediastinal and pulmonary vasculature

Helical scanning has provided new techniques for non-invasive demonstration of thoracic and mediastinal vessels by optimising contrast media enhancement.[15,21]

CT angiography is indicated for:

- Thoracic aortic aneurysm/dissection[21] replacing an aortogram in the writer's department.

- Superior vena cava (SVC) obstruction.[6]

- Detection of pulmonary thromboemboli in segmental pulmonary vessels.[15] Pulmonary angiography is still seen as the 'gold standard' investigation but, it is invasive.

- Arteriovenous malformation.[2,6]

- Aortic graft assessment.[6]

An enhanced scan will demonstrate the vasculature and any abnormality. Comparison with an unenhanced scan may provide additional information and should be performed first if indicated. The acquired data can be used to reconstruct overlapping slices for 3D, MP reformats, SSD and MIPs, to add to the information obtained. There appears to be little benefit to 'over-reconstructing'[8] - experience endorses this – although other sources suggest more is better.[22] In practice, in the writer's department, an average of 2–3 reconstructions per slice thickness appears to provide optimum image manipulation. While 3D reformatting and SSD can provide the surgeon with a 'road-map' and additional viewpoints, the extra diagnostic information they provide, however, is limited.[6,21] CT angiography is not, as yet, an examination of choice for cardiac investigations. The fast helical acquisition is still not fast enough to capture the heart at rest and, even with movement reduction algorithms, some blurring occurs.

Table 4.1 – Scan parameters for CT angiography of the mediastinal and pulmonary vasculature.

Beam collimation	5–7 mm
Reconstruction interval	2–7 mm
Pitch	1.5–2, to allow a single breath hold
Standard algorithm	Lung/detail or bone algorithm if appropriate
Matrix	512
kVp	120[8]
mA	200[8]
Imaging	Mediastinal settings, lung settings if appropriate

Protocol for CT angiography

A routine unenhanced thorax scan may be performed first, if necessary. The area should be planned to cover from above to below the vessels of interest, with a reduced FOV as appropriate. The details of the protocol are given in Table 4.1.

For contrast 100 ml of IV contrast media, 200 mg iodine/ml, is injected (usually at the ante-cubital vein) using a pump injector. A lower concentration of contrast media is used to avoid artefact from a dense bolus of contrast.

For SVC obstruction (Figures 4.26 and 4.27) injecting through both right and left arms simultaneously, i.e. 50 ml of contrast media through each, can greatly improve demonstration of the vessels involved with any

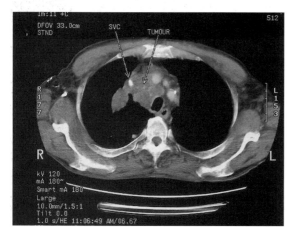

Figure 4.26 — IV contrast-enhanced thorax scan demonstrating superior vena cava (SVC) surrounded by tumour.

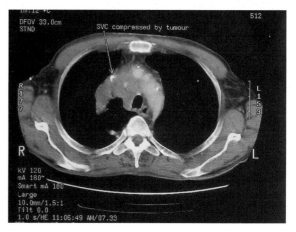

Figure 4.27 — IV contrast thorax scan demonstrating tumour obstructing SVC.

obstruction; this reduces dilution of the contrast medium by unenhanced blood from the other arm. However, it may be impracticable.

The rate of injection and the scan delays depend upon the structures to be demonstrated. Suggested injection rates and scan delays are shown in Table 4.2. Alternatively a method of monitoring contrast density, in order to scan at peak enhancement may be used. Some scanner manufacturers include this as part of the software, e.g. 'Smart prep'.[23] Figures 4.28 and 4.29 show contrast-enhanced mediastinum scans and the anatomy that can be demonstrated.

MP reformats, obtained from overlapping reconstructed images, are shown in Figures 4.30–4.32. A beam collimation of 5mm was used for acquisition and the raw data were reconstructed with a 3mm interval.

Dissecting aortic aneurysm: a note of caution

A word of warning: it is possible with helical CT to miss a dissecting aortic aneurysm. This is because there may be a discrepancy in the contrast bolus filling both the false and true lumen at the same time and therefore the flap may not be clearly demonstrated. To avoid this, either the scan can be repeated almost immediately without any further contrast, or it may be better to revert to conventional dynamic scanning, with a few contiguous slices or a very short helical scan repeated at intervals through the region of interest.

High resolution CT for lung parenchyma

This is indicated for:

- interstitial lung disease
- bronchiectasis, airway disease[17]
- differentiation of focal lung disease[12]
- differentiation of pulmonary nodules[12]

A routine thorax scan is not indicated here, since it is only the lung parenchyma in fine detail that is important. Incremental conventional slice by slice scanning is used to acquire thin slices of data, reconstructed using a lung or bone algorithm. They may be clustered together for shorter scanning times if the equipment allows. Depending upon the clinical question, it may be possible to limit the scan to the area or levels of interest. These thin slices, together with the selection of a small pixel size, produce images with the high spatial resolution necessary for demonstrating lung structure (Figure 4.33). The very thin slices reduce the partial volume effect providing detailed demonstration of small pulmonary nodules or lesions.[5] ROI measurements may assist in nodule differentiation.

Protocol for high-resolution CT for lung parenchyma

The patient is in the supine position, although it may be of advantage to position the patient prone since the

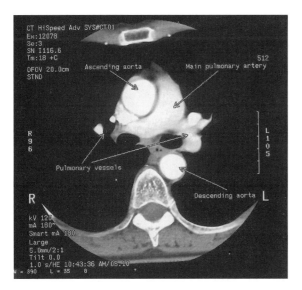

Figure 4.28 — CT angiography demonstrating mediastinal great vessels.

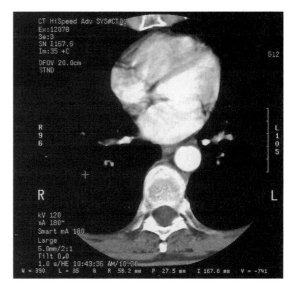

Figure 4.29 — CT angiography demonstrating heart, descending aorta and pulmonary vessels.

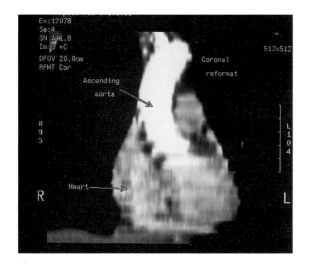

Figure 4.30 — Coronal reformat using data from IV contrast thorax scan; demonstrating heart and great vessels.

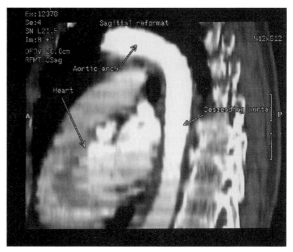

Figure 4.31 — Sagittal reformat demonstrating heart and great vessels.

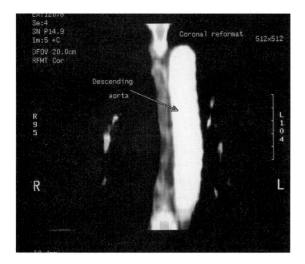

Figure 4.32 — Coronal reformat demonstrating descending aorta.

'ground glass' appearance which can occur with interstitial lung disease may be confused with fluid in the lung bases if the patient is supine. However, it may not be possible for the patient to lie prone but, regardless of position, the patient should be made as comfortable as possible.

The patient may go head or feet first through the gantry.

The patient is centred, using laser centring lights, to the sternal notch if supine and to the spinous process of C7 if prone, in the midline and to the mid-axillary line.

The arms are raised above the head. Further details of the protocol are given in Table 4.3.

This type of scan can be seen in Figure 4.33.

Limited thin slice helical CT for areas of interest

This is indicated for:

- differentiation of focal lung disease[6]
- differentiation of pulmonary nodules[6]
- airway disease[17]
- bone pathology

A routine thorax scan is usually necessary, initially to localise the area of interest and to aid planning for the limited thin slices.

Table 4.2 – Suggested injection rates and scan delays in CT angiography of the mediastinal and pulmonary vasculature

Area under examination	Injection rate, ml/s	Scan delay, sec
Mediastinum	2	30
Ascending aorta	4–5	15–20
Descending aorta	3	25–30
Pulmonary vessels	5	15
SVC obstruction	2	15–20

Table 4.3 – Scan parameters for high-resolution CT for lung parenchyma

Beam collimation	1–3 mm
Table increment	10 mm, to include from the apices to the base of the lungs, or selectively through levels of interest
Respiration	Suspended; scans clustered together if possible, for reduced number of breath-holds
Algorithm	Lung/detail or bone algorithm only
Matrix	512
Field of view (FOV)	
Scan	Dependent upon patient size
Display	Dependent upon area to be scanned
kVp	120[8]
mA	100–200[8]
Scan time	1 sec[8]
Imaging	Lung settings only, 1550 WW and –550 WL

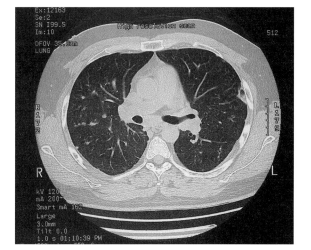

Figure 4.33 — High resolution thorax scan 3mm beam collimation acquired at 10mm increments using a lung algorithm only. Lung parenchyma is demonstrated with higher resolution than with scans acquired using the routine thorax protocol; comparison can be made with Figure 4.6.

Protocol for limited thin slice helical CT

Protocol parameters are given in Table 4.4. This type of scan can be seen in Figure 4.34. ROI measurements can be made to assist with lesion or nodule differentiation and contrast enhancement may be used to compare the ROIs pre and post contrast. However the most accurate method of determining tissue type is by histological investigation of a biopsy sample.

Alternatively the volume data acquired for the routine scan may be retrospectively reconstructed through the area of interest, using different algorithms, a smaller FOV and with a smaller reconstruction interval, as appropriate. However, this may not give enough detail since the data would have been acquired using a wide beam collimation; compare Figure 4.1 with Figure 4.34.

Interventional CT of the thorax

This may be diagnostic, as in biopsy of tissue, or therapeutic, as in aspiration or drainage. It is safer and less costly than surgical intervention.[24] The protocol would be similar for either situation.

The necessity of CT guidance should have been ascertained previously, since other imaging modalities such as ultrasound or fluoroscopy, may be adequate and reduce the patient's radiation exposure.

Table 4.4 – Scan parameters for limited thin slice helical CT

Beam collimation	1–3 mm
Reconstruction interval	1–3 mm
Pitch	1–1.5
Respiration	Suspended; usually a single breath-hold
Algorithm	Dependent on area under examination
Matrix	512
kVp	120[8]
mA	200[8]
FOV	Limited to cover the area of interest; planned from the routine scan
Imaging	Appropriate settings for the tissue to be demonstrated

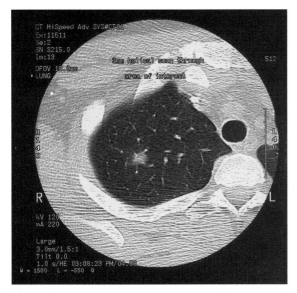

Figure 4.34 — A 3mm helical slice acquired with a 3mm reconstruction interval. Centred over the area of interest for lesion differentiation. Comparison can be made with Figure 4.1.

A diagnostic CT scan may have already been performed necessitating only limited low-dose scans to localise the area for biopsy or aspiration. The procedure is usually performed by a radiologist.

The patient's consent should be obtained for this interventional procedure after they have been informed of the possible risks involved such as that of a pneumothorax.

Protocol for interventional thoracic CT

Patient preparation and explanation is essential for these procedures to be performed safely. It is extremely important that the patient keeps still during the procedure, since the slightest movement can jeopardise the accuracy of the localisation measurements. An extra few minutes spent making the patient comfortable and explaining breath-holding techniques will benefit all concerned.

The patient should be positioned to allow the radiologist the easiest access to the area under examination.

A scout view is useful for planning the localising scans or it may be possible to plan from the diagnostic scans.

A limited helical acquisition or contiguous slices through the area of interest are adequate. The beam collimation selected should be suitable for the area of interest (usually 5–10 mm) but wide enough for easy localisation of the needle tip. The FOV should be large enough to include skin surfaces in order to accurately measure the entry point for the biopsy or aspiration needle and the distance from skin to area of examination.

The phase of respiration should be the same for all scans throughout the procedure. This should be explained to the patient prior to the examination. The scan can be performed using the most appropriate algorithm for tissue type, with image windows to demonstrate the area of examination to the best advantage. These scans are for guidance only.

Exposure factors and all other scanning parameters are similar to a diagnostic scan.

Accurate measurements can be made using a radiolucent skin marker, attached to the patient's skin prior to scanning, as a reference point. Alternatively, most scanning software includes a grid which can be displayed over the localisation slice, corresponding with the laser centring lights and enabling an accurate and simple method of measuring. Figure 4.35 shows both a radiolucent skin marker and measuring grid.

Once the appropriate slice for biopsy or aspiration has been agreed, this level should be noted, and localising measurements obtained from this scan. These should include:

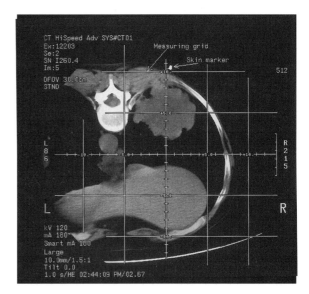

Figure 4.35. — Biopsy measurements can be made using a grid or a radiolucent skin marker; both are demonstrated here.

1. A measurement from the skin marker to the preferred point of needle entry or from the grid line which corresponds to the laser centring light.

2. A measurement from the preferred point of needle entry to the area under examination (Figure 4.36).

The patient is then moved into the position of the selected slice level, which is marked on the skin using a waterproof marker. At this level the localisation measurements should be clearly and accurately marked. These measurements should be checked with the radiologist performing the protocol.

The biopsy or aspiration should be carried out using an aseptic technique and equipment according to the departmental procedure.

Two or three helical or contiguous scans may be necessary to locate the needle tip, performed at intervals during the procedure centred, on the needle, using scan exposures and parameters similar to the planning scan. Once the needle tip is in position, a biopsy sample or aspirate can be obtained and sent for laboratory investigations. Alternatively a drain may be sited.

Depending on departmental protocol, it may be necessary to repeat the scans through the area under examination, to ensure the patient does not have a pneumothorax, or a chest X-ray may be requested. Figure 4.37 shows a pneumothorax caused at biopsy of a lesion.

The procedure should be documented with token images. A suggested selection is as follows:

- a scout view with a reference line indicating the level of biopsy or aspiration
- a scan showing the measurements and level of scan
- a scan showing the needle tip or drain in position
- a check scan demonstrating presence or absence of a pneumothorax

At the end of the procedure the patient should be observed, according to departmental protocol, but in any case ensuring regular checks on the entry site and patient's breathing. Interventional techniques can vary between radiologists and departments; the most important features are aseptic technique and accurate measurements for localisation.

Radiotherapy planning

A mention should be made of the part played by CT in aiding the radiotherapy department to plan treatment to the thorax for their patients. Although CT simulators are available, planning can be a lengthy procedure using them. CT provides the radiotherapist with information about the cross-sectional anatomy of the patient, which is very important when planning treatment. Using these cross-sectional images, care can be taken to avoid sensitive structures being damaged by the radiation dose.

In general conventional slice by slice imaging is used, because it is thought that the interpolation algorithms used in helical CT do not as yet provide enough accuracy for radiotherapy (RT) planning. However,

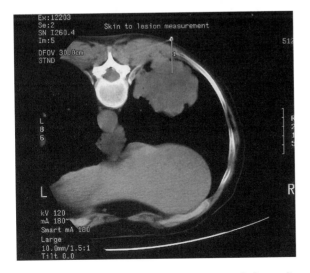

Figure 4.36. — Biopsy localisation measurement made from radiolucent skin marker to lesion.

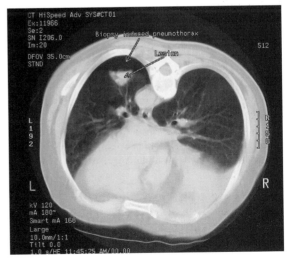

Figure 4.37 — Pneumothorax caused by biopsy needle.

improving technology will probably overcome this and bring the advantages of helical CT to the radiotherapy patient in the future.

The planning scan usually involves a scout view to include radiolucent skin markers positioned prior to scanning.

The patient has to be positioned exactly as for radiotherapy treatment. This usually means that a rigid table top must replace the soft mattress used on most scanners, and various restraints are used to keep the patient in a precise position.

The scan slices are contiguous, with a beam collimation suitable for the area to be treated; this is usually 5–10 mm. The FOV has to be large enough to include skin surfaces and radiolucent markers (Figure 4.38). The scan parameters are similar to those for a routine thorax scan, except for suspended respiration; the latter cannot be simulated for the duration of the radiotherapy treatment.

Once the area to be treated has been identified on the scan slices, the treatment fields are marked on the patient's skin using indelible ink and guided by the laser centring lights.

Where systems allow the scan information is then networked to the radiotherapy department in order to plan the patient's treatment.

Conclusion

CT scanning has long been accepted as an excellent imaging modality for demonstrating thoracic patholo-

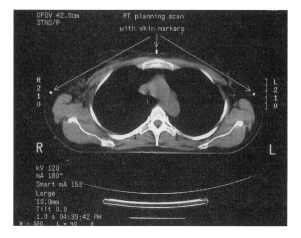

Figure 4.38 — Radiotherapy planning scan; large field of view to include skin markers.

gy. Helical scanning techniques have vastly improved the quality of CT scanning of the thorax, enabling single breath-hold imaging, capturing particular phases of vascular enhancement and generally increasing the amount of information available from a single CT scan. The cost of that information, however, is a radiation dose much greater than that of a chest X-ray and so CT should only be requested when the clinical question cannot be answered elsewhere. For the patient it has brought the benefits of a quick, simple, non-invasive diagnostic test.

This chapter has attempted to provide a standard routine protocol for CT scanning of the thorax, largely employing helical techniques. The details are not meant to have been 'carved in stone' but to be used as a guide or starting block from where it is possible to supplement or tailor the procedure to suit the situation and answer the clinical question posed.

References

1. Flower CDR Williams MP. The pleural space. In: Husband JES, (ed.) *CT Review.* New York: Churchill Livingstone, 1989; 23–32.

2. Costello P. Thorax. In: Zeman RK *et al.*, (ed.) *Helical/spiral CT: a practical approach.* New York: McGraw-Hill, 1995; 105–152.

3. Royal College of Radiologists. *The use of CT in the initial investigation of common malignancies.* 1994.

4. Kalender WA. Seissler W Klotz E. Spiral volumetric CT with single-breath-hold technique, continuous transport and continuous scanner rotation. *Radiology* 1990; **176**: 181–183.

5. Seeram E. *Computed tomography: physical principles, clinical applications and quality control.* Philadelphia: WB. Saunders,. 1994; 110–123, 198–218, 166–181.

6. Brink JA. McFarland EG, Heiken JP. Review: helical/spiral computed body tomography. *Clin Radiol* 1997; **52**: 489–503.

7. Kalender WA., Polacin A. Physical performance characteristics of spiral CT scanning. *Med Phys* 1991; **18** (5): 914.

8. GE. Medical Systems. Personal communication. Bracknell, 1997.

9. Cann CE. Quantitative accuracy of spiral versus discrete volume CT scanning [abstract]. *Radiology* 1992; **85**: 126–127.

10. Remy-Jardin M. Remy J., Giraud F., Marquette CH. Pulmonary nodules: detection with thick section spiral CT versus conventional CT. *Radiology* 1993; **187**: 513–520.

11. Kalender WA. Technical foundations of spiral CT. *Semin Ultrasound CT MRI.* 1994; **15** (2): 81–89.

12. Dixon AK. *Body CT, A handbook.* London: Churchill Livingstone,. 1983; 98–112.

13. Rogalla P., Mutze S., Hamm B. *Body CT: state of the art.* Munich: W Zuckschwerdt Verlag,. 1996; xii.

14. Glazer HS. Differential diagnosis of mediastinal pathology. In: Husband JES (ed.) *CT Review.* New York: Churchill Livingstone, 1989; 41–51.

15. Remy-Jardin M Remy J Wattine L Giraud F. Central pulmonary thromboembolism: diagnosis with spiral volumetric CT with the single breath-hold technique – comparison with pulmonary angiography. *Radiology* 1992; **185**: 381–387.

16. Goodman LR., Lipchick RJ. Diagnosis of acute pulmonary embolism: time for a new approach. *Radiology* 1996; **199**: 25–27.

17. Costello P. Spiral CT of the thorax. *Semin Ultrasound, CT MRI* 1994; **15**(2): 90–106.

18. Flower CDR. Williams MP. Staging bronchial cancer. In: Husband JES.(ed.) *CT Review*. New York: Churchill Livingstone, 1989; 13–21.

19. Glazer HS. CT of pulmonary collapse. In: Husband JES, (ed.) *CT Review*. New York: Churchill Livingstone, 1989: 33–40.

20. Edwards CRW Bouchier IAD. *Davidson's principles and practice of medicine*. (16th edn.) New York: Churchill Livingstone, 1993; 898–899.

21. Quint LE *et al*. Evaluation of thoracic aortic disease with the use of helical CT and multiplanar reconstructions: Comparison with surgical findings. *Radiology* 1996; **201**: 37–41.

22. Kalender WA., Polacin A., Suss C. A comparison of conventional and spiral CT: an experimental study on the detection of spherical lesions. *J Comput Axial Tomogr* 1994; **18**: 167–176

23. GE. Medical Systems. *CT HiSpeed Advantage technical reference*. Operator's reference 2: 74 Paris 1995.

24. Dunnick NR. Interventional CT. In: Husband JES, (ed). *CT Review*. New York: Churchill Livingstone, 1989; 179–190.

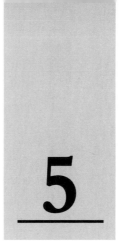

5

CONTRAST ENHANCEMENT IN CT

Peter Dawson

Introduction

Contrast is a photographic term or, more precisely, in the present context, a radiographic term, which denotes the difference in appearance in an image between one anatomical region and another, or between a region of abnormality and the surrounding normal tissue. The latter is sometimes referred to as lesion conspicuity. In plain film radiography, natural soft tissue contrast resolution is poor and it is for this reason that contrast-enhancing agents for oral and intravascular use were developed in the first place.

The introduction of CT brought with it an enormous advance over plain films in soft tissue contrast resolution but, nevertheless, even CT greatly benefits from artificial pharmacological contrast enhancement by oral, rectal and intravascular routes. In this chapter we will concentrate on the use of intravascular contrast agents.

The basic parameter in a CT image is the 'CT number' (CT N°). The CT N° is defined with respect to water X-ray absorption and over an (arbitrary) scale of –1000 to +1000.

$$CT\ N° = \frac{\text{Absorption coefficient} - \text{absorption coefficient water}}{\text{Absorption coefficient water}} \times 1000$$

With fast scanning the CT N° may be measured at frequent intervals and curves generated (Figure 5.1). Radiographic contrast in the CT image is a function of the fractional difference in CT N° between two regions or between the abnormal and the normal (conspicuity):

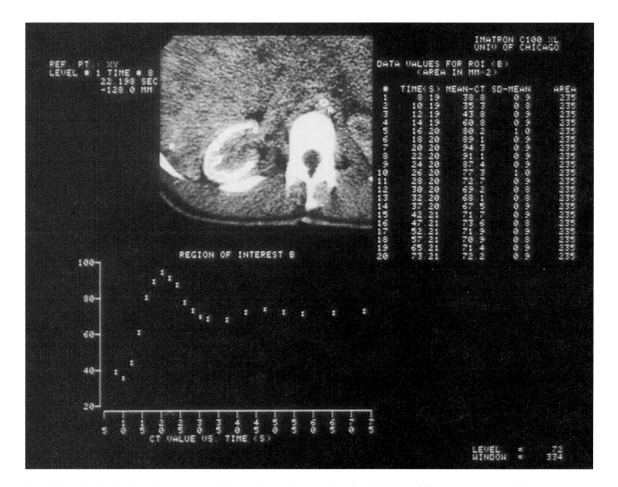

Figure 5.1 — A plot of CT N° (pre contrast CT N° subtracted) versus time for the kidney, following intravenous bolus contrast agent administration.

$$\text{Conspicuity} = \text{CT N}° \text{ abnormal} - \text{CT N}° \text{ normal}$$

In practice, 'contrast enhancement' is a term frequently used to describe the generalised increase in CT N° by the giving of an intravenous contrast agent. Strictly speaking, an increase in CT N° in, say, the liver may be little different in normal and abnormal regions, resulting in no increased lesion conspicuity. In short 'contrast enhancement' in the loose sense does not always lead to the desired contrast enhancement of the image. Conspicuity of lesions may actually, on occasion, decrease following administration of contrast agent. If a hypodense lesion enhances more than its normal surrounding then it may become isodense with consequent loss of conspicuity. The factors dictating such effects are complex, but may be understood without too much difficulty if a few simplifications are made.

Contrast agents are usually given intravenously into an antecubital vein but, on occasion, may be given into a lower limb vein or even intra-arterially as will be discussed later. Injection rates prescribed by different departments and individuals vary a great deal, even to the extent that there is confusion about what constitutes a 'bolus' and what constitutes an 'infusion'. Before tackling these issues, it is essential to discuss the basic pharmacokinetics of the agents.

Contrast agents

Intravascular contrast agents are injectable solutions of X-ray absorbing materials. The X-ray absorbing factor could, in principle, be a variety of elements but iodine is universally used in all the commercial formulations.

The chemistry of the agents has been well documented and will not be repeated here.[1] In brief, the agents are based on the tri-iodated benzene ring (Figure 5.2). Commercial products come in a number of formulations and strengths. We will not be concerned here with any pharmacological effects which are also well documented elsewhere,[2] but will deal exclusively with their pharmacokinetics since it is these which dictate the distribution and concentrations in the body at any time after injection and which, therefore, dictate contrast enhancement.

Pharmacokinetics

All contrast agents are small molecules which, consequently, rather freely cross endothelial membranes,[3] except in the brain where the blood-brain barrier prevents this. They do not enter cells to any significant degree, and so distribute themselves in the whole extracellular fluid space, intra- and extravascular. They are sometimes described as extracellular fluid space markers. They are excreted exclusively by the kidneys by passive glomerular filtration with no active tubular reabsorption or secretion.[4]

Following injection by any intravascular route, a bolus is rapidly diluted in the circulating plasma, leaks into the extravascular space and begins filtration in the kidneys. All the events happen simultaneously, making the detailed mathematical description of events in the first minute or so dauntingly complex and difficult.[3] Indeed, even much of the basic pharmacological data necessary for a detailed analysis has, surprisingly, not been collected.[3] All experimental work has concentrated on the later pharmacokinetics.[4,5] Unfortunately, this early

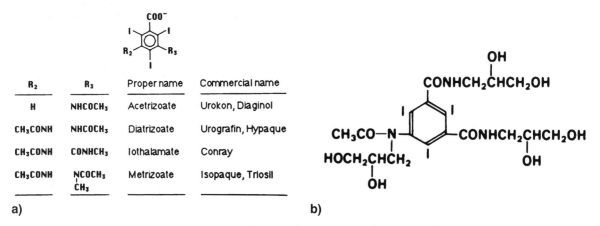

R₂	R₃	Proper name	Commercial name
H	NHCOCH₃	Acetrizoate	Urokon, Diaginol
CH₃CONH	NHCOCH₃	Diatrizoate	Urografin, Hypaque
CH₃CONH	CONHCH₃	Iothalamate	Conray
CH₃CONH	NCOCH₃ CH₃	Metrizoate	Isopaque, Triosil

a)

b)

Figure 5.2 — Some iodinated X-ray contrast agents. Both are based on an iodinated benzene ring skeleton. a) Ionic monomeric agents (several manufacturers). b) Non-ionic monomeric agents iohexol (Omnipaque; – Nycomed, Oslo, Norway).

period is what is frequently of greatest interest in an era of fast scanners. The usual two-compartment model[5] which describes the distribution of contrast between plasma (compartment 1) and interstitium (compartment 2), (Figure 5.3), is entirely anatomically appropriate, but an assumption is made that there is complete mixing in the circulating plasma before leak into the interstitium and renal filtration are allowed to begin. This makes possible a useful analysis of later pharmacokinetics, but is irrelevant to most CT enhancement.

In this chapter we will attempt only a qualitatively descriptive approach to the subject, but in sufficient detail as to allow a proper appreciation of events. We start with some obvious and simple facts and build up a more complete picture progressively.

- If a contrast agent is injected intravenously in a bolus it will take some 10 seconds, depending on cardiac output, to reach the systemic arterial circulation and will arrive diluted and with some having leaked out of the circulation during transit. From this point onwards contrast will appear in the arterial circulation of the organs and tissues of interest.

- For a rapid bolus injection, the contrast concentration-time curve in an observed artery will have a height and width dependent on the cardiac output.[3] Poor cardiac output will mean a lower peak and a greater width for any particular bolus. This is intuitively obvious. If the contrast agent were trickled extremely slowly into a peripheral vein one would not expect a high peaked, narrow and short-lived contrast bolus to appear on the arterial side.

- Imaging at this stage (very early) will allow arteries to be well visualised: CT arteriography.

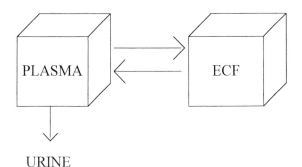

Figure 5.3 — The two-compartment model of contrast agent pharmacokinetics and distribution. The two compartments are plasma and interstitium (extravascular extracellular space).

- A rapid and brief intravenous bolus will pass quite quickly, even with poor cardiac output, so a brief scan of a few slices, or a spiral scan of a small volume, may well miss such a contrast bolus. Hence the use in practice of slower, more prolonged infusions. However, for the moment we will continue to consider bolus injections for simplicity.

- A few seconds later, a parenchymogram will appear. This is due to contrast agent throughout the whole capillary bed of the organ and to contrast agent leaked out, even at first pass, into the interstitial space. In the brain, the blood–brain barrier prevents such a leak when there is no pathology to impair it, and the enhancement of the normal brain is entirely due to contrast agent in blood vessels.

Because of dilution in the circulating blood and loss by leak to interstitium, blood levels peak early and decline rapidly. Interstitial levels rise more slowly and fall later. Early on, blood levels exceed interstitial levels; later, interstitial concentrations exceed blood concentrations. The cross-over point occurs at varying times in different tissues and is called the equilibrium point.[6,7] All times after this equilibrium point are said to be in the equilibrium phase, a phase usually avoided in scanning as discussed later. Note that the arterial curve time course can be monitored by sampling a large vessel such as the aorta, but the interstitial curve cannot be followed at all, since any region of interest chosen will contain both interstitium and small blood vessels. There is no way of directly monitoring interstitial concentrations of contrast. When we sample a region of interest in the tissue and obtain a CT N° time curve, we are looking at contrast medium both in vessels and in interstitium, the precise proportion between the two varying with tissue.[6,7] If we plot a tissue curve with an arterial curve, the result is typically as in (Figure 5.4). These curves do not cross and the precise equilibrium point and beginning of the equilibrium phase is difficult to discern. Note that the suggestion frequently made in the literature to the effect that it is the phase in which these curves become parallel is incorrect. In general these curves will not be parallel. The equilibrium phase may be thought of roughly as the phase in which they decline together.[6]

This is the basic picture on which all the following development of an understanding of contrast enhancement may be built. Increase in the CT N° of a tissue is a function of blood vessel and interstitial contrast concentrations. Relative concentrations in these compartments are a function of time and of the precise capillary permeability (this is always high but is, nevertheless,

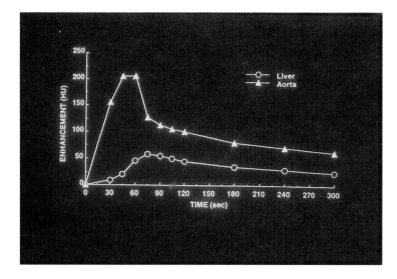

Figure 5.4 — Typical aortic and tissue curves (liver in this case). Note that the tissue curve is not an interstitial curve but a combination of interstitial and blood curves in the region of interest, The curves do not cross and, contrary to statements in the literature, do not (quite) become parallel.

variable).[3] The increase in the CT N° will also depend on the proportion of the volume of the region of interest (ROI) which is blood vessel and the proportion which is interstitium.[6] For example, if the blood vessel concentrations are very high, but only, say, 1% of a rather avascular tissue is blood vessels, then the enhancement effect will not be high and vice versa. Similarly, for varying proportionate volumes of interstitium. Qualitatively at least, these arguments are easy to develop and follow. They may be expressed mathematically, but this approach will not be pursued here.

It is obvious that, details aside, enhancement, in the sense of an increase of overall CT N°, will rise to a peak and decline over a variable period. However, that the conspicuity of an abnormality, say a tumour, in a tissue will be enhanced is not obviously guaranteed. If the tumour behaves in much the same way as the normal tissue, then no useful change in conspicuity is to be expected. Even though the whole tissue 'enhances', if a tumour has a similar proportionate vascularity, proportionate interstitial volume and proportionate cellular volume and if it contains blood vessels which are of a similar permeability to the normal tissue, then it will exhibit much the same enhancement pattern as that normal tissue and 'contrast enhancement' will offer little in the way of improvement in conspicuity. Obviously, in practice, abnormalities almost by definition, exhibit variations from the normal range in multiple structural parameters and so different behaviour is, in general, to be expected. In other words, improvements in conspicuity are, on the whole to be expected when a contrast agent is given. Nevertheless, even having said this, it must be remembered that there may still be phases of the enhancement during which this will be more or less true or not true at all. For this reason many favour scanning during more than one phase of enhancement to minimise the danger of such a loss of information. This becomes a practical option with modern fast scanners.

We will now try to apply these principles to the enhancement of the liver, this organ being chosen for two reasons. Firstly, it is one of the most important organs in CT scanning. Secondly, it presents a particularly important and complex challenge because of its dual circulation. Thirdly, notwithstanding this extra complexity, the early phase of its enhancement (hepatic arterial) follows just the same pattern as is found in any other organ. It is particularly useful therefore to rehearse all the facts we have assembled in the context of liver imaging.

Liver enhancement

Hepatic arterial phase

Following a peripheral venous injection, contrast agent arrives after, say, 10 seconds, depending on cardiac output, in the aorta and thence the hepatic artery. Since normal liver gains only some 15% of its blood supply from the hepatic artery, it will only enhance modestly during this phase. Liver tumours on the other hand, obtain 85% of their blood supply from hepatic artery and may enhance significantly in this early phase. Indeed, some particularly vascular tumours may enhance more brightly than normal liver at this stage. However, the typical liver lesion, starting as hypodense with respect to the normal liver will often enhance more than the normal liver and become isodense. That is to say conspicuity may be lost. Very early scanning is necessary to observe this phase and it may actually be useful to carry it out in the case, say, of suspected metastases from particularly vascular tumours such as pancreatic neuro-endocrine tumours as these may transiently become hyperdense. Care is generally required, however, as more information may be lost than gained, as discussed.

This phase may be better seen and exploited by inserting a catheter directly into the common hepatic artery in the angiography suite and transferring the patient to the CT suite with the catheter in situ. Direct injection of contrast in this manner is called CT hepatic arteriography.[8,9] It is only performed occasionally, but may be very useful in the patient with suspected hypervascular metastases.

Portal venal phase

As contrast arrives in the hepatic artery, it also arrives in the splenic artery, (Figure 5,5a), the superior mesenteric, (Figure 5.5b), and the inferior mesenteric arteries. Some 10 seconds later still, it returns via the splenic, (Figure 5.6a), superior mesenteric, (Figure 5.6b), and inferior mesenteric veins to fill the portal vein. Since normal liver obtains some 85% of its blood supply by this route, marked normal liver enhancement is seen in this phase. Tumours, on the other hand, which obtain only 15% of their blood supply by this route enhance

relatively poorly, even if 'vascular'. In this phase, such tumours are likely to become hypodense with respect to normal liver again. Note that there may again be a short period of loss of conspicuity in the case of a hypervascular lesion, (having become hyperdense during the hepatic arterial phase) as the normal liver catches it up but before it overtakes the lesion.

Again, this portal venous phase may be better exploited by placing a catheter appropriately, with the patient in the angiography suite. It is not possible routinely to catheterise the portal vein directly and so a catheter is placed either in the superior mesenteric artery (SMA) or into the splenic artery. When the patient has been transferred to the CT suite, injection of contrast into either of these arteries produces a venous return of contrast in the portal vein at a much higher concentration than can be achieved by peripheral venous injection. This is CT arterioportography.[10,11] Note that if imaging is too long delayed following this injection, then the advantages of the technique may be lost as contrast returns via the hepatic veins to the inferior vena cava, (IVC), the right heart, the lungs and the left heart and systemic circulation and, albeit in diluted form, to the aorta and hepatic artery. Hepatic arterial enhancement of tumour may then diminish the contrast between tumour and normal liver which was achieved earlier in the true portal venous phase.

Practical applications

So far we have discussed the principles of intravascular contrast administration without considering specific

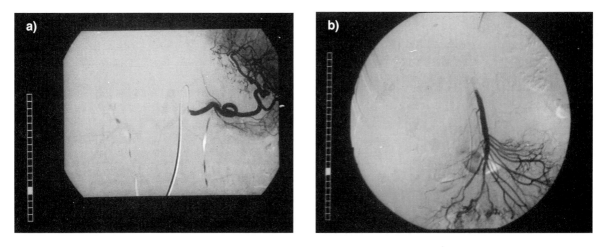

Figure 5.5 — a) Splenic, and b) superior mesenteric arteriograms. Contrast arrives in these vessels alnost simultaneously following IV injection.

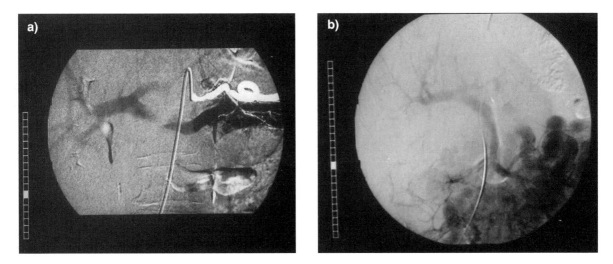

Figure 5.6 — The venous phases of Figure 5.5. Contrast returns in the a) splenic and b) superior mesenteric veins to fill the portal venous system. In the former case the portal vein is extrinsically compressed.

concentrations and administration rate regimes. The point has already been made that a rapid bolus is not usually appropriate for use with fast scanning, since it is obvious that the required phase might simply be missed. Usually, a slower, more prolonged injection/ infusion is given to obviate this difficulty. It is self-evident that such regimes may lead to the simultaneous realisation of different phases of enhancement. For example, contrast agent may still be reaching the hepatic artery while earlier contrast agent is already in the portal vein.

Some illustrative clinical examples

LABELLING OF BLOOD VESSELS

It is useful to enhance blood vessels with contrast agent simply in order to 'label' them and distinguish them from other structures. To achieve this end alone, no special regime or timing are required. An example of this is shown in Figure 5.7.

CT ARTERIOGRAPHY

Spiral scanning allows a volume data set to be obtained which may be used for good quality three dimensional reconstructions, (see for example, Figure 5.8).

CT (ARTERIO) PORTOGRAPHY

Like CT arteriography this is a demanding technique in a number of ways, requiring the use of both CT and angiography suites and both CT and angiographic per-

sonnel. A catheter is placed in the SMA or splenic artery and the liver is scanned while contrast is infusing the portal vein (normal liver). Figure 5.9 illustrates a typical result. A tumour deposit is seen as a non-enhancing region within the enhancing liver, as discussed above. Higher sections show contrast medium in hepatic veins, which also assists in the delineation of liver segmental anatomies. Later, the filling of the systemic arteries represents a potential danger to the examination in that the tumour, fed by hepatic artery, may enhance sufficiently as to become isodense with normal liver and be lost.

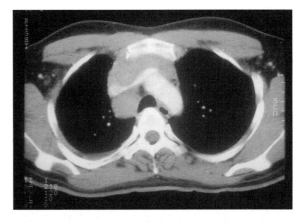

Figure 5.7 — Contrast in blood vessels, in this case in the innominate vein, SVC and aortic arch differentiates vessels from mediastinal mass.

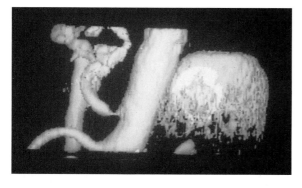

Figure 5.8 — A single projection from a 3D reconstruction from a spiral (helical) volume data set. There is a stenosis in the coeliac axis.

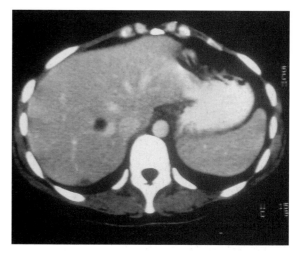

THE ROUTINE PERIPHERAL VENOUS INJECTION

Figure 5.10a illustrates a vascular lesion in the liver well demonstrated during the arterial phase when it enhances markedly. Figure 5.10b demonstrates the potential danger of scanning at the wrong time. The lesion disappears in the later portal phase. Modern fast scanners allow images to be obtained in several phases of enhancement, reducing such dangers.

TISSUE CHARACTERISATION

Unfortunately, there is little in the unenhanced CT appearances in most lesions to indicate their character. A cyst or cystic component may be recognised and a high fat content similarly detected. The presence of calcification is another possible indicator of nature, but much beyond this it is not possible to go.

Figure 5.9 — An image from a CT portogram. Contrast is injected into the superior mesenteric artery (or splenic artery) and scanning takes place as the contrast returns in the portal vein to enhance normal liver. The tumour, being supplied primarily by the hepatic artery, does not enhance and is consequently seen as a 'filling defect'. The image is late in the sequence, as may be deduced from the presence of contrast in the aorta.

Given that the pattern of enhancement of a lesion is a function of aspects of its structure, such as proportionate vascular, proportionate interstitial and proportionate cellular volumes, and of capillary permeability, it might reasonably be hoped that details of enhancement patterns might give at least some strong pointers to the nature of the lesion. Unfortunately, this has been found not to be the case except in a small handful of

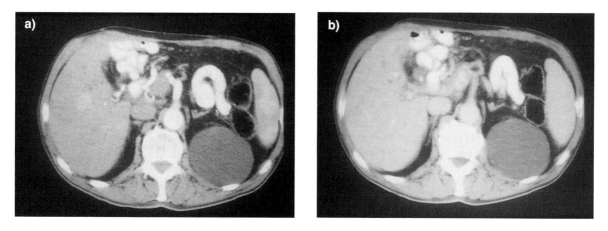

Figure 5.10 — a) A lesion well seen during the hepatic arterial phase following IV injection. b) This lesion subsequently disappears in the portal venous phase

exceptions – for example, the cerebral abscess with its classical peripheral rim enhancement and the cavernous haemangioma of the liver which, classically, exhibits a characteristic 'filling in' from the periphery to the centre. Actually, the true characteristic finding here is not so much of the 'filling in' but the fact that, at any stage, the enhancement in the lesion is the same as that seen in blood vessels, Figure 5.11. The reason for this is that the contrast agent in the lesion is largely in large vascular spaces.

QUANTITATIVE MEASUREMENTS

CT numbers have a distinctive and useful property. If the pre-contrast – background CT number is subtracted, the CT number in a region of interest at any time is reliably proportional to the contrast concentrations.[12] This has been successfully exploited to derive physiological data such as tissue perfusion and, in the kidney, glomerular filtration rate (GFR), from the CT number – time curves obtained in dynamic scans following bolus injection.

This is a potentially important new field, but is beyond the scope of this chapter.[13]

Summary

Contrast enhancement in CT is a complex and time-dependent phenomenon, but may readily be understood in general terms on the basis of a handful of simple facts about contrast agent pharmacokinetics. Armed with a simple analysis, it becomes possible to understand contrast enhancement strategies. Having said this, the reader is advised that if the great variety of recommended contrast agent dose and administration regimes seems to suggest that there is confusion among radiologists. The author would be inclined to reply to the effect: 'you might say that; I could not possibly comment'.

References

1. Dawson P. Water soluble contrast media. In : Whitehouse GM, Worthington BJ (eds). *Techniques in diagnostic imaging.* Blackwell Scientific, 1995,

2. Dawson P. Chemotoxicity of contrast media and clinical adverse effects; a review. *Investigative Radiol* 1985; **20**: 52–59.

3. Blomley MJK, Dawson P. Bolus dynamics: theoretical and experimental aspects. *Br J Radiol* 1997; **70**: 351–359.

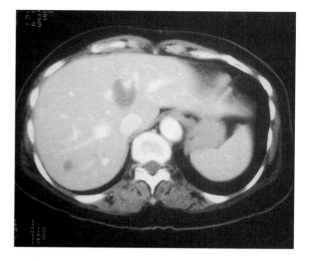

Figure 5.11 — The characteristic enhancement pattern of a liver cavernous haemangioma. The hallmark is not 'filling in' from the periphery which may, in any case, be incomplete, but more the fact that the peripheral nodular rim enhancement matches the blood vessel enhancement at any stage.

4. Dawson P. Glomerular filtration rate determined using contrast clearance: should we all be doing it? *Curr Opin* Urol 1996; **6**: 75–77.

5. Blomley MJK, Dawson P. The quantification of renal function with enhanced computed tomography. [review] *Br J of Radiol* 1996; **69**: 989–995

6. Dawson P, Blomley MJK Contrast agents pharmacokinetics revisited. I Reformulation. *Acad Radiol* 1996; **3**: S261-S263.

7. Blomley MJK, Dawson P. Contrast agent pharmacokinetics revisited. II Computer aided analysis. *Acad Radiol* 1996; **3**: S264-S267.

8. Moss AA, Dean PB, Axel I. Dynamic CT of hepatic masses with intravenous and intra-arterial contrast material. *Am J of Roentgenol* 1982; **138**: 847–852.

9. Oudkerk M, Van Ooijen B, Mali SPM. Liver metastases from colorectal carcinoma. Detection with continuous CT angiography. *Radiology* 1992; **185**: 157–161.

10. Matsul 0, Takashima T, Kadoya M. Liver metastases from colorectal cancers: Detection with CT during arterial portography. *Radiology* 1987; **165**: 65–69.

11. Miller DL, Simmons JT, Chang R. Hepatic metastasis detection: Comparison of three CT contrast enhancement methods. *Radiology* 1987; **165**: 785–796.

12. Dean PB, Plewes DB. Contrast media in computed tomography. In: Sovak M (ed) *Radiocontrast agents* Berlin: Springer Verlag, 1984,

13. Dawson P, Blomley MJK, Cosgrove DO. Functional and physiological imaging. In: Grainger RG, Allison DJA (eds): *Diagnostic Radiology: A Textbook of Medical Imaging*, 3rd edn Churchill Livingstone, 1996,

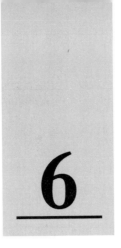

6

THE ABDOMEN

Sheila Rankin

Technique

The main technical details for abdominal survey are summarised in Box 6.1

Box 6.1 — TECHNIQUE FOR ABDOMINAL SURVEY

- Oral contrast
- Collimation: 8–10 mm scans through the abdomen
- Contiguous scans through organ of interest
- Non contiguous scans can be used for retro-peritoneal adenopathy
- Intravenous contrast if required
- Appropriate field of view

Oral contrast

In routine abdominal scanning patients are given oral contrast to opacify the bowel and allow differentiation from adjacent pathological lesions. In most instances patients are given 800 ml of positive oral contrast, either a dilute barium suspension (E-Z-CAT, E-Z-EM), or a 3% solution of gastrografin (sodium/meglumine diatrizoate. Schering) or similar water-soluble contrast which may be flavoured with fruit squash. The contrast is given 30–40 minutes before the scan to opacify the small bowel and a further 200 ml of the same contrast is given immediately before the scan to opacify the stomach and proximal small bowel.

Although positive contrast is used in routine scanning, if the stomach is the primary organ of interest, for instance in the staging of gastric cancer, water can be used as a negative contrast to improve visualisation of the gastric wall, the patient being given 400 ml to drink immediately prior to the scan. Do not mix the two protocols as the visualisation of the gastric wall is then very poor as it becomes isodense with the oral contrast. A similar contrast regime may be used for the pancreas.

To opacify the colon two doses of contrast are given: 800 ml of oral contrast the night before the scan to fill the colon and a second 800 ml to opacify the small bowel, given as usual before the scan. Alternatively, rectal contrast (using 200 ml of 6% water-soluble contrast) can be given immediately before the scan to opacify the rectum and sigmoid. If the colon is the organ of interest, for example in performing a CT enema for the diagnosis of colonic cancer, the patient can be given bowel preparation followed by a muscle relaxant (Buscopan,scopolamine butylbromide) and air insufflation to distend the colon, but no rectal contrast is required.

Intravenous contrast

The use of contrast (see Chapter 5) is at the discretion of the radiologist. Intravenous contrast may be used to opacify the vessels and aid their differentiation from retroperitoneal nodes. It is also frequently used to characterise liver lesions (p. 74), renal masses and pancreatic disease and in the assessment of the aorta. Unenhanced scans may be performed with the post contrast scans targeted to a specific organ, or a post contrast scan only may be performed, which will decrease the radiation dose to the patient. The timing of the administration of the contrast may be critical particularly with the modern spiral or helical CT scanners.

Slice thickness (collimation)

For survey scans a slice thickness of 8–10 mm is used, depending on the type of scanner. Contiguous scans are used through an area of interest; however noncontiguous scans, with a consequent decrease in patient dose, may be taken through the retroperitoneum when assessing nodal disease, with no loss of diagnostic quality. This is because only lymph nodes greater than 1 cm in short axis diameter are considered abnormal, so it is not significant if 5 mm of the patient is not scanned and a 5 mm node missed.

To improve spatial resolution 3–5 mm collimation should be used for specific organs particularly if small lesions are to be identified. If thinner collimation is used the mA value must be increased to decrease noise which limits resolution. Generally 1 mm collimation cannot be used in the body because the noise is prohibitive.

Field of view

All of the patient should be included in the initial field of view and the image then reconstructed with a targeted field of view. This will improve spatial resolution as the pixel size will be decreased (remembering that pixel size = field of view/matrix). This is particularly important for organs such as the pancreas and aorta where a 250 mm field of view is optimal, although the full field of view may also be required to assess the remainder of the abdomen.

Spiral/helical CT

In conventional CT single slices are obtained with a stationary table, whereas in spiral/helical CT[1,2] continuous rotation of the tube and detector system in one direction is possible (see Chapter 1, p. 3). The development of higher output X-ray tubes capable of producing continuous radiation for up to 100 seconds combined with continuous table movement, produces a volume of data that looks like a spiral or helix, rather than individual slices.

The two main limitations in body CT scanning are:

1. Respiratory misregistration: when the patient takes a different breath hold for each scan so that areas may be either scanned twice or missed completely.

2. Partial volume effect: when a lesion is only partially contained within a slice, leading to averaging of CT numbers within the voxel of the lesion and the surrounding structures and thus inaccurate attenuation values. This is a particular problem in the liver and kidneys where cysts may be mistaken for solid lesions based on CT numbers.

The development of spiral CT allows the chest or abdomen to be scanned on a single breath hold, thus eliminating respiratory misregistration. The scans can be reconstructed anywhere within the scanned volume so one can find the slice that is optimally positioned to minimise the partial volume effect for a lesion. For lesions smaller than the chosen slice thickness the only solution is to rescan using thinner collimation.

Spiral scans provide optimal imaging of contrast in organs as the scans can be performed rapidly at peak opacification. It is therefore very important that the contrast is delivered at the appropriate time in relation to the scan.

For multiplanar reformats (MPR) and 3D imaging, spiral data allows the production of multiple overlapping slices and, consequently, greatly improved final images with no increase in radiation to the patient.

Technical factors

Slip rings – These may be ' high voltage' when the required voltage is passed across the slip rings to the tube or ' low voltage ' when a low voltage goes across the slip rings and is stepped up in the gantry.

X-ray tubes – These continue to be improved so that higher mA values may be maintained for longer periods. This has resulted in tubes of up to 6.5 million heat units and improved cooling rates of more than 1 million units/minute. The mA value in spiral CT is less than in conventional scans, particularly if long exposures are used. This may be a problem with very large patients and some compromises between scan duration and mA value is required.

Scan time – This ranges between 0.75 and 2 seconds per rotation. Most machines scan at 1 second.

Detectors – Improved detector efficiency is also important as the mA values may be limited, and both gas and solid state detectors are used.

Performance

Dose - The dose per mA is the same as with a conventional scan. However the mA value used may be lower, so there is a decrease in dose. When the scans are acquired for 2D and 3D imaging, as overlapping slices are generated from the acquired volume without additional irradiation, there may be considerable reduction in overall patient dose.

Noise – In the original spiral CT scanners, using 360° interpolation of data, for a given mA value noise was reduced, compared to a conventional scan, by a factor of 0.82. The data are now reconstructed using 180° interpolation which increases noise by 12–29%. In addition the mA value used in spiral CT may be less than in conventional CT so generally spiral scans are noisier than conventional scans.

Effective slice thickness - As the table is moving continuously during the data acquisition there is some z axis blur with an increase in effective slice thickness but the new reconstruction algorithms, using 180° rather than 360° interpolation, minimise this.

Z-axis blurring – The full-width half-maximum (FWHM) is about 1.1 wider than a conventional scan using 180° interpolation and even with a pitch of 2 it is only increased by a factor of 1.3. For example using a pitch of 2 the FWHM of a nominal 5 mm slice is 6.4 mm.[3] This can potentially increase the problem of the partial volume effect, but this is overcome by the ability to reconstruct the data at any given position.

Tube heating – The mA that can be produced with a spiral scan is about 90% of the value that can be produced by a 1 second conventional scan. However as the number of rotations increases the maximal allowed mA will decrease.

Computers – Increased computational power means more raw data can be stored so back-to-back spirals can be performed, and rapid, almost real-time, processing of data is available on some of the newer scanners. Additional software produced by some manufacturers allows dose reduction by computing the most appropriate mA value to be used, based on the patient's size, and also the most appropriate time to commence scanning after intravenous contrast has been given.

Operator choices

In spiral CT the distance covered by a scan depends on the slice thickness (collimation), the duration of the scan and the table feed speed. The duration of a spiral scan ranges between 24 and 100 seconds depending on the type of scanner and protocols may require modification to take account of this.

The ratio of the collimation and the table feed speed is the pitch. In general a pitch of 1 (where slice thickness in mm = table feed in mm/sec) is best as this produces minimal z axis blur. However to cover the volume of interest a pitch of up to 2 may be required. A pitch of 2 is the maximum available. Using thinner collimation with a pitch greater than 1 will produces a smaller effective slice thickness than using the next slice thickness available with a pitch of 1, but will cover the same distance. For example using a 3 mm slice with a pitch of 1.67 (3 mm slice, table moves at 5 mm per second) gives an effective slice thickness of 3.8 mm, as opposed to a 5 mm slice with a pitch of 1(5 mm slice, table moves at 5 mm per second) which gives an effective slice thickness of 5.2 mm. Both these protocols would cover the same distance for a given number of rotations.

Intravenous contrast: timing and volume

The amount and timing of the contrast injection is vital. Many centres use non-ionic contrast at a concentration of 300 mg/ml.

In vascular imaging the length of the bolus should equal the scan duration to maximise contrast levels, using an injection rate of between 3 and 6 ml/sec. The volume to be injected is calculated by multiplying the injection rate by the scan duration. The timing of the delay between the onset of the injection and commencing the scan is very important, to ensure optimal contrast in the vessel of interest.

For non-vascular imaging the volume and timing of contrast administration varies depending on the organ of interest.

Reconstruction

In spiral CT the scans can be reconstructed anywhere along the volume to produce overlapping slices, with no increase in radiation. Longitudinal resolution improves when the reconstruction interval is less than the collimation, but only to a certain level and reconstructing two images per rotation is recommended to improve lesion detection and reconstruction of three images per rotation will produce better 3D images.

Spiral imaging: the major decisions

These are as follows:

1. *Maximum duration of the breath hold*. Most patients can hold their breath for 30 seconds particularly if they are hyperventilated prior to the scan.

2. *Slice width*: This should be the thinnest value possible to improve spatial resolution, with the maximum mA value possible to minimise noise.

3. *Distance* to be covered by the scan.

4. *Pitch*: This should be as close to 1 as possible, to cover the distance required and minimise z axis blur, however it is often better to use a pitch of 2 and thinner collimation than a larger slice width and a pitch of 1. The pitch may be variable or a fixed ratio depending on the scanner. The first parameter to define is the table speed, and from this the compromise between pitch and slice thickness is calculated.

$$\text{Table speed} = \frac{\text{Required scan length (distance)}}{\text{Tolerable breath hold}}$$

$$\text{Pitch} = \frac{\text{Table speed Gantry rotation period(s)}}{\text{Slice width}}$$

For example if the distance to be covered by the scan is 250 mm and the patient can hold their breath for 25 seconds the table speed is 10 mm/second. Thus the slice thickness could be 10 mm with a pitch of 1 or, for better spatial resolution, a 5 mm slice with a pitch of 2, assuming a 1 second scan time.

5. *Contrast:* If this is to be used for vascular imaging the bolus should equal the scan length to maximise contrast (see above).

Volume of contrast used = Injection rate × scan duration

6. *Reconstruction index* As previously mentioned in spiral CT the scans can be reconstructed anywhere along the volume to give overlapping slices. An overlap of 50% is recommended to improve lesion detection and produce better 3D images. Obviously every

available slice could be reconstructed but this is time consuming and produces no discernible improvement in the quality of the 3D images. Reconstruction of overlapping slices requires raw data.

7. *Field of View (FOV).* Use a targeted field of view, as the decrease in the size of pixel will increase the resolution. However for multiplanar reformats, if the entire scan is to be included, as it is reconstructed as a cube, the FOV should be the same as the table travel.

A low noise reconstruction kernel (smooth) may be better for 2D and 3D imaging.

8. *Post processing of the data.* The main programs used to produce 2D and 3D images involve curved or linear multiplanar reconstructions (MPR), surface shaded display (SSD), maximum intensity projections (MIP) and volume rendering (not available on all workstations).

Many units are now replacing their older scanners with spiral/helical CT and suggested protocols for spiral scanning will be stressed, particularly if they differ significantly from conventional scanning.

Stomach

The stomach is a distensible structure and when it is collapsed the lumen is obscured. The normal gastric wall is 3–5 mm thick. In order to assess gastric wall thickening, which occurs with gastric cancer and lymphoma, the stomach must be fully distended. This can be achieved by giving an extra 200 ml of contrast immediately prior to the scan with or without the use of gas-producing agents and positioning the patient so as to optimally distend any questionable areas. If the stomach is the primary organ of interest the use of negative contrast (water) is suggested (Figure 6.1).

To accurately stage gastric cancer, the primary tumour and extension into adjacent organs and the presence of involved lymph nodes must be assessed. The following technique is suggested when using a spiral scanner. It can be modified slightly for dynamic incremental scanning.

1. To adequately distend the stomach, 20 mg of Buscopan (scopolamine butylbromide) is given intramuscularly 5 minutes before the scan, assuming there are no contraindications. The Buscopan decreases the artefacts from peristalsis and delays gastric emptying.

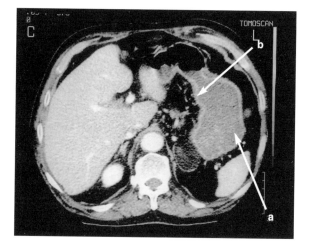

Figure 6.1 — Stomach wall well visualised when water is used as negative contrast a, water filled gastric lumen; b, gastric wall.

2. Immediately prior the scan, 400 ml of water is drunk to distend the stomach.

3. Intravenous contrast,100 ml is given at a rate of 3 ml/sec.

4. Scanning is commenced 40 sec after the administration of contrast has begun.

5. Collimation of 5 mm is used. Coeliac and left gastric nodes are considered abnormal if greater than 8 mm; therefore, to adequately identify them a thinner collimation than that used for a normal abdominal survey is required. This protocol is more sensitive for identifying both the primary tumour and involved lymph nodes than conventional scanning using 10 mm collimation. [4]

Pancreas

Anatomy of the pancreas

The long axis of the body of the pancreas lies obliquely across the spine with the tail adjacent to the splenic hilus. The neck lies anterior to the junction of the superior mesenteric vein and the splenic vein forming the portal vein, with the head and uncinate process extending inferiorly. The splenic vein lies posterior to the body and tail and the most inferior portion of the pancreas (uncinate process) is identified anterior to the junction of the left renal vein and inferior vena cava. The head measures 2 cm, the neck 1 cm and the body and tail 1–2 cm. The pancreatic duct will be seen in up to 75% of patients if thin section 3–5 mm collimation is used, and especially if intravenous contrast is given as the normal pancreas enhances, accentuating the difference between the gland and low attenuation duct. The common bile duct (3–6 mm) will normally be identified within the pancreatic head close to the lateral and posterior wall. The main pancreatic duct (1–3 mm) lies parallel and medial to the common bile duct (Figure 6.2).

The normal unenhanced pancreas has CT numbers of 30–40 Hounsfield units (HU) and enhances homogeneously to 100–150 HU after a bolus of contrast (100–180 ml). To optimise this enhancement, the delay between the onset of the injection and the scanning depends whether a conventional scanner (30–40 second delay) or a spiral scanner (45–60 second delay) is used. The larger volume of contrast is needed with a conventional scanner as incremental dynamic scanning is slower than spiral scanning and the scan should be performed at peak pancreatic enhancement which will need to be maintained for a longer period for conventional scanning.

There is normally a fat plane between the pancreas and the superior mesenteric artery, but not between the neck of the pancreas and the portal vein. The pancreas may be smooth or lobulated in outline and fatty replacement of the pancreas may be seen in the elderly.

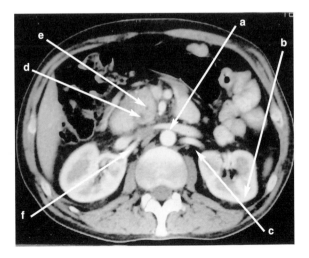

Figure 6.2 — Scan through the head and uncinate process of the pancreas a, left renal vein; b, left kidney with excellent corticomedullary differentiation; c, left renal artery; d, common bile duct; e, pancreatic duct; f, right renal artery.

Clinical applications of CT in pancreatic disease

These include:

1. Acute pancreatitis

2. Chronic pancreatitis

3. Diagnosis and staging of pancreatic tumours.

ACUTE PANCREATITIS. (Box 6.2)

CT is used to demonstrate morphological changes in pancreatitis and to identify complications that may require intervention.

In 30 % of patients with acute pancreatitis the CT scan will be normal. The changes that may be seen include diffuse or focal gland enlargement, peripancreatic inflammatory changes and fluid collections which may extend into the mediastinum, along the root of the mesentery, around the caecum and into the pelvis.

Pancreatic viability is assessed using the post contrast scan which should always be performed. Pancreatic necrosis develops early in severe acute pancreatitis, and there is good correlation between the identification of pancreatic necrosis and the development of complications and death, with patient morbidity of 94% and mortality of 29% if there is necrosis of over 30% of the pancreas.[5] Pancreatic necrosis is defined as a diffuse or focal area of non-viable parenchyma and appears as a diffuse or well marginated area of unenhanced pancreatic parenchyma on a post contrast CT scan (Figure 6.3). CT is 80–90% accurate in the detection of pancreatic necrosis.

Pancreatic abscesses, which usually occur 4 weeks after the acute event, are thick-walled collections

---

Box 6.2 — TECHNIQUE FOR PANCREATITIS

- Oral contrast
- Unenhanced 8–10 mm scans through the abdomen to identify pancreas and any fluid collections
- Post contrast 5 mm scans through the pancreas to assess pancreatic viability
- Incremental dynamic scanning, 30–40 sec delay
- spiral scanning, 45–60 sec delay
- Contrast injection 100–180 ml at 3 ml/sec, to visualise pancreas at peak enhancement

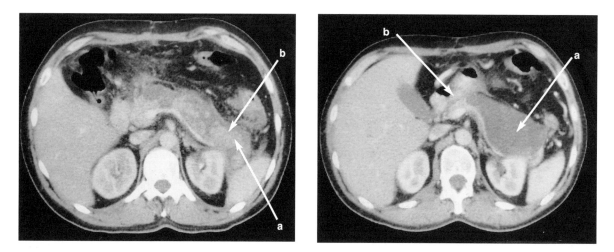

Figure 6.3 — CT of acute pancreatitis with pancreatic necrosis. a) a, Normal enhancement of the pancreas; b, necrotic non enhanced pancreatic tissue. b) Three weeks later. No viable pancreatic tissue in body or tail (a); small amount of viable enhancing pancreatic neck (b).

which may contain gas bubbles. They are treated by percutaneous drainage, whereas infected pancreatic necrosis, which carries a much higher mortality, requires surgical intervention.

CHRONIC PANCREATITIS

The main features of chronic pancreatitis are pancreatic duct dilatation, parenchymal atrophy and pancreatic calcification, all of which are well seen on CT. Thin section 3–5 mm collimation should be used to optimise visualisation of duct abnormalities: in one study[6] ductal abnormalities were identified in 88% of patients, and the missed cases were those in which only 10 mm slices were used.

To optimise the visualisation of pancreatic calcification, negative bowel contrast (water) may be advantageous. Fatty replacement of the pancreas is readily visualised as a decrease in the normal pancreatic attenuation and fibrosis and inflammatory infiltrates are identified as areas of inhomogeneous enhancement, however mild changes can be missed on CT.

PANCREATIC NEOPLASMS

Adenocarcinoma – This accounts for 90% of pancreatic tumours and CT will detect approximately 95% of these tumours. The majority (60%) occur in the head of the pancreas and present with biliary duct obstruction, 15% arise in the body and 5% in the tail; in 20% the gland is diffusely involved. The tumours in the body and tail present later and are larger at the time of diag-

nosis. On unenhanced scans the attenuation of the carcinoma is very similar to that of the normal pancreas, and thus tumours will only be identified when they are large enough to focally distort the pancreatic contour. Following intravenous contrast most carcinomas enhance less than the normal pancreas, especially when there are high circulating levels of contrast, and small carcinomas which do not distort the contour can be identified, particularly if thin collimation (3–5 mm) is used. In patients with acute or chronic pancreatitis focal areas of decreased perfusion may occur and carcinoma and pancreatitis can co-exist, if there is any doubt about the diagnosis CT guided percutaneous biopsy can be undertaken.

Staging – Pancreatic carcinoma is often advanced at time of presentation with only 14% of patients having tumour limited to the pancreas; 65% will have advanced local disease or disseminated distant metastases, and 21% will have localised disease involving regional lymph nodes. Surgery offers the only cure but will not be undertaken if there are hepatic metastases, involved lymph nodes beyond the resection field or vascular encasement. Therefore, to adequately stage patients, intravenous contrast is given to identify liver metastases and vascular invasion. Vascular invasion is diagnosed if there is loss of the fat plane around the mesenteric vessels or if there is an obvious change in calibre of the coeliac artery, mesenteric vessels or portal vein (Figure 6.4). Dilatation of pancreatico-duodenal veins has recently been described as an additional finding in unresectable pancreatic cancer.[7]

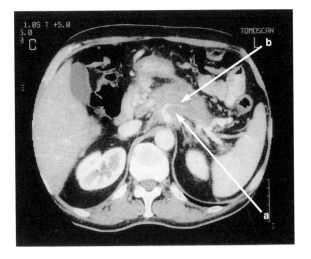

Figure 6.4 — CT scan of pancreatic carcinoma of the body (a), with vascular invasion and narrowing of the splenic artery (b).

Technique – The scanning technique using incremental dynamic scanning is similar to that for acute pancreatitis, making sure the liver is included and using the larger volume of contrast.

A technique for spiral CT is suggested below in Box 6.3. If the patient cannot hold their breath long enough for the entire liver and pancreas to be scanned on a single breath-hold then the pancreas is scanned with 3–5 mm collimation and the remainder of the liver with 7–10 mm collimation. This may also be used if the length of spiral required is not available, so 2 back to

---

Box 6.3 — TECHNIQUE FOR SPIRAL CT IN PANCREATIC CANCER

- Oral contrast (water)
- Unenhanced 8–10 mm scans to identify the limits of the pancreas
- Collimation 3 mm; pitch of 1.6
  or
- Collimation 5 mm; pitch of 1
- Scan from bottom of pancreas upwards to include the liver
- Change to 7–10 mm slice, if necessary, to complete the coverage of the liver
- Contrast injected, 100–150 ml at 3 ml/sec
- Delay 50–60 seconds

---

back spirals must be obtained. When changing from one technique to another there is usually a 7–9 second delay during which time the patient breathes. The whole scan should take approximately 40 seconds and the liver can be scanned at peak hepatic enhancement to diagnose any metastases. Overlapping reconstructions can be obtained through the pancreas which may aid the identification of vascular invasion.

Islet cell Tumours – Islet tumours, which are hypervascular tumours may be either functioning or non-functioning (15%). Non-functioning tumours are larger at the time of diagnosis and usually present with metastases. The functioning tumours are small, and all are hypervascular compared to the remainder of the pancreas and calcification is present in 20%. These tumours are more likely to be identified if narrow collimation and overlapping slices are generated and if the pancreas is scanned in the arterial phase of contrast enhancement (delay of 30 seconds). Spiral technology allows dual phase scanning, in an early arterial phase and a later parenchymal phase which may improve tumour detection. The liver metastases are also hypervascular and may be better identified if the liver is scanned in the hepatic arterial phase (20–30 second delay), rather than the portal venous phase (60 second delay).

Kidneys

Anatomy of the kidneys

The kidneys and adrenal glands are surrounded by an envelope of fat and lie within the renal fascia. Posteriorly the renal fascia is well defined and is continuous with the lateral conal fascia which lies lateral to the ascending or descending colon. The posterior fascia is laminated and fluid may track within it. The anterior renal fascia which merges with the posterior fascia to form the lateral conal fascia, is the posterior boundary of the anterior pararenal space which contains the pancreas, ascending and descending colon and most of the duodenum. The anterior renal fascia is frequently thickened secondary to inflammation of the pancreas or colon. The perirenal space contains the kidneys, adrenals, renal vessels and proximal ureters and surrounding fat.

The cross sectional anatomy of the kidney is easily identified on CT as the surrounding fat provides contrast. The posterior and anterior surfaces are seen in their entirety. On unenhanced scans the CT number of the renal cortex is 30–60 HU. The renal pelvis can usually be identified as water density but the calices are not normally seen. The renal vein lying anterior to the artery at the renal hilum is easily visualised. Intravenous contrast is required to fully assess the kidney. The aorta, renal artery and vein opacify 20–30 seconds after the contrast is injected followed by the corticomedullary phase at 50 seconds (Figure 6.2) and the nephrogram phase at 100–180 seconds. The CT number of the cortex will increase to 80–120 HU and is maximal in the corticomedullary phase; however the medullary attenuation may be greater in the nephrogram phase. Contrast then passes into the calices and pelvis at 3–4 minutes after injection.

In conventional CT there may be incomplete renal imaging because of the mobility of the kidney. The advent of spiral CT, allowing the acquisition of a volume of data with no respiratory misregistration, has greatly improved renal visualisation. Scans can also be performed during the rapid administration of a bolus of contrast, so contrast levels are high throughout the scan and thus good arterial, corticomedullary, nephrogram and caliceal images may be obtained. In addition multiple overlapping slices can be obtained with no increase in radiation, and thus superb 2D and 3D images may be generated from the acquired data.

Clinical applications of CT in renal conditions

These include:

1. Assessment of renal masses and differentiation of solid and cystic lesions.
2. Tumour staging and surgical planning.
3. Renal trauma.
4. Non-invasive diagnosis of renal artery stenosis.
5. Renal colic.

Technique for CT scanning of kidneys

The details are summarised in Box 6.4. The following issues are also important.

1. *Precontrast scans* for the position of the kidneys are made, to identify calcification and to obtain accurate precontrast attenuation values of masses.
2. *Contrast:* 90–120 ml of 300 mg/ml injected at 3 ml/s.
3. *Post contrast scans* if using incremental dynamic scanning, 5 mm collimation with a 40 second delay.
4. *Spiral scanner* If this is used, the slice collimation depends on the patient's ability to hold their breath

---

> **Box 6.4 — TECHNIQUE FOR KIDNEYS**
>
> - Oral contrast
> - Unenhanced 8–10 mm scans through the kidneys to identify calcification and obtain attenuation values of any renal masses
> - Contrast 100 ml intravenously at 3 ml/sec
> - Post contrast 5 mm scans through the kidneys
> - Incremental dynamic scanning, 30–40 second delay
> - Spiral scanning, 45–180 second delay; scan from the bottom up
> - Include the liver if staging malignancy; may require two spirals for optimal timing

and the distance to be covered to include both kidneys. Usually a 5 mm slice with a pitch of 1 (table speed 5 mm/sec) and reconstruction every 3 mm is used. A thinner slice of 3 mm and a pitch of 1.5–2 may be advantageous, especially if very small lesions are to be assessed. However if the patient is large, weighing more than 100 kg, a 5 mm slice should be used as there is a limit to the mA value that is available and the images may be very noisy. [9]

5. *Scan delay* depends on whether corticomedullary images (50 second delay) or nephrogram images (100–180 second delay) are required. Small renal lesions are usually better seen on nephrogram images, but renal perfusion is better assessed on corticomedullary images. Delayed scans at 5 minutes allow assessment of caliceal detail. Back-to-back spirals may allow both assessment of the renal veins and inferior vena cava and the maximum conspicuity of small renal lesions. [10]

Assessment of renal masses

RENAL CYSTS

The commonest renal mass in an adult is a cyst. The CT characteristics of a benign cyst are are follows:

1. Homogeneous and of water density, CT number 0–20 HU.
2. No enhancement after contrast
3. No detectable wall where cyst projects outside the renal outline
4. Smooth interface with the parenchyma.

If the lesion exhibits all these features, no further investigation is required. If the mass is very small, partial volume averaging may give an erroneously high CT number, so it is important to use thin collimation. Some cysts may be hyperdense and may require further investigation with ultrasound or percutaneous aspiration. Cysts which have thick walls or calcification are indeterminate masses; these may represent cystic tumours and will require further assessment.

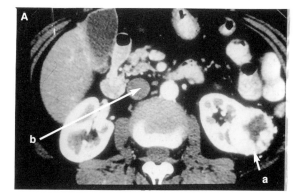

RENAL CELL CARCINOMA

Renal cell carcinoma accounts for 85% of all renal malignancy, and 30% of the patients will have metastases at the time of presentation.

The characteristics of renal cell carcinoma include the following:

1. A heterogeneous mass with attenuation less than normal kidney.
2. Enhancement following contrast, but normally less than the surrounding renal tissue on delayed scans. On early arterial phase scans, vascular staining may be seen.
3. Irregular interface with renal parenchyma.
4. If a wall is present, it is thick and irregular.
5. Secondary signs:
   — renal vein or inferior vena caval invasion by tumour
   — lymph node enlargement
   — extracapsular spread of tumour
   — tumour calcification
   — distant metastases.

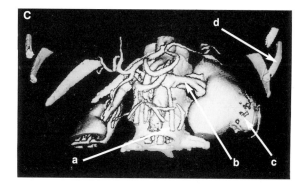

TUMOUR STAGING

The technique for the primary tumour can be as described in Box 6.4. When using a spiral scanner the optimal time for identifying renal masses is in the nephrogram phase, i.e. after a 120–180 second delay, but this is suboptimal for either the liver or the renal veins. Therefore one could perform two separate investigations, one to diagnose and another to stage the tumour. However in many cases the diagnosis of renal cell cancer has already been made on ultrasound and a compromise is made. To look for renal vein involvement early scans (30 second delay) may be best; however a potential pitfall is the flow artefact seen in the supra-renal inferior vena cava (IVC) when opacified blood from the renal veins is mixed with non opacified blood from the infrarenal IVC and this may mimic thrombus (Figure 6.5a and b). To assess the liver for metastases a delay of 60 seconds is best, and this allows further assessment of the IVC. Therefore it is probably

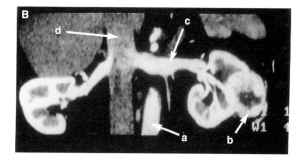

Figure 6.5 — A: CT scan of renal cell cancer (a). Unopacified blood from the legs in the inferior vena cava (IVC) (b) as the scan has been taken below the level of the renal veins. B: Coronal reformat through the kidneys. a, contrast in aorta;. b, renal cell cancer; c, left renal vein containing contrast; d, suprarenal IVC with a mixture of contrast enhanced blood from the renal veins and unopacified blood from the legs. (see also Figure 6.10.) C: 3D Surface shaded display of kidneys, to aid surgical planning. a, left gonadal vein; b, left renal vein; c, left renal tumour; d, ribs (Figure 6.5 is reproduced by kind permission of Professor Reznek, St Bartholomew's Hospital, London).

better to scan from the bottom up so that the liver is scanned at an optimal time. Alternatively many of the newer scanners can do back to back spirals thus allowing two or three spirals to be performed with different timing to provide superb visualisation of the renal vein, kidney and liver on a single examination.

Surgical planning

Surgeons may wish to perform nephron-sparing surgery, and the ability to produce excellent 2D and 3D images helps the planning of partial nephrectomies. To produce the necessary image quality a 3–5 mm collimation and a pitch of 1 is suggested. Many surgeons prefer to look at the 3D surface shaded display which can be rotated to simulate operative orientation (Figure 6.5c).

Renal trauma

Spiral scanning is ideally suited for patients with abdominal trauma, as it allows the rapid acquisition of data in critically ill patients at optimal vascular opacification.

In general, in abdominal scanning following trauma, precontrast scans are not usually performed. Oral contrast is administered if possible. A delay of 45–60 seconds between injection and the commencement of scanning will allow assessment of parenchymal perfusion defects in the liver, spleen and kidneys and the diagnosis of arterial extravasation. There will be no contrast within the calices, so calcification within the collecting system can be identified. Delayed scans at 10 minutes will be required to assess the integrity of the caliceal system if the patient's condition permits. Either 8–10 mm collimation with a pitch of 1, or 5 mm collimation and a pitch of 1.5–2 can be used depending on the size of the patient and the ability to hold their breath. If necessary the scans through the pelvis can be done using a conventional non spiral mode.

Renal artery stenosis

Spiral CT can be used in hypertensive patients to assess the renal arteries non invasively, to exclude renal artery stenosis and also for the preoperative assessment of liver related renal donors to document arterial anatomy that may influence surgery.[11] Significant renal artery stenosis (>70%) can be diagnosed by spiral CT. In one series[12] all patients with renal artery stenosis were identified but 4 out of 22

were graded incorrectly based on axial images only; the addition of curved MP reformats and 3D rendering resulted in all studies being diagnostic. Rubin and colleagues[13] found maximum intensity projection to be more sensitive and accurate than surface shaded display (SSD) for stenosis greater than 70%. Surface shaded display is less accurate because calcification is not visualised separately from contrast and stenoses may be underestimated, and partial volume averaging will be accentuated by the thresholding process and arterial discontinuity may be created.

CT also has the advantage that it may identify other causes for the hypertension, such as adrenal tumours. Recent studies by Cochran et al[11] found that CT angiography was as accurate as conventional angiography in the preoperative assessment of liver related renal donors, with a considerable reduction in the cost.

SUGGESTED TECHNIQUE.

1. *Scanogram*

2. *Precontrast.* A 5 mm scan from the diaphragms to at least 6 cm below the origin of the superior mesenteric artery, to identify the adrenals, localise the renal arteries and assess the required distance to be covered by the spiral, and a 10 mm scan to the aortic bifurcation to exclude an aortic aneurysm, are performed.

3. *Cardiac output estimate.* Here, a 5 mm slice just above renal arteries, and a dynamic multislice technique with no table movement are employed. Inject 10–15 ml of contrast at 4 ml/sec. After an 8 second delay, scans are done every 2 seconds (i.e. there is a 2 second interscan delay). Use low mA and kV values to reduce the dose to the patient and the heat loading on the tube. Plot time-density curves of the enhancement of the aorta, or 'eyeball' the scan with the maximum enhancement, to work out the delay (time to maximum enhancement +8 sec) then add 3 seconds to allow for a larger volume of injected contrast. Alternatively one can use the software provided on some scanners to start scanning at an appropriate time.

4. *Diagnostic scan.* Use a 3 mm slice and a pitch of 1 and reconstruct every 1 mm, or use a 2 mm slice, pitch of 1–1.5 (depending on the distance to be covered) and reconstruct every 1 mm.

Renal colic

Recently, spiral CT has been used to investigate patients with suspected renal colic. Unenhanced scans

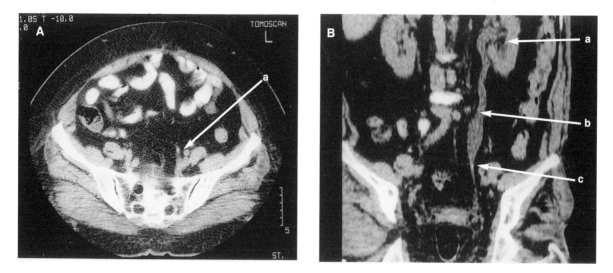

Figure 6.6 — A: Axial scan through the pelvis showing small renal calculus (a). B: Coronal reformat showing dilated ureter above the calculus a, left kidney; b, dilated left ureter; c, ureteric calculus.

covering the entire renal tract can be performed so renal calculi can be identified. Using a 5 mm slice with a pitch of 2 and reconstruction every 3 mm will allow the abdomen and pelvis to be included on a single spiral and good quality reformatted images to be obtained (Figure 6.6). If necessary back-to-back spirals can be performed for instance, if the patient can only hold their breath for a limited time or if there is a limited tube output. Sommer *et al*[14] found spiral CT to be more sensitive than ultrasound combined with an abdominal film in the detection of ureteric calculi, and Smith *et al*[15] found CT to be better than intravenous urography for ureteric stones and equally good for diagnosing obstruction. Furthermore CT has the advantage that other causes of abdominal pain may also be identified.

CT angiography

The advent of spiral CT has revolutionised non-invasive methods of assessing the vascular tree.[16,17] CT can be used for the preoperative assessment of aortic aneurysms for both surgery and stent insertion (Figure 6.7). It is less invasive than angiography and more accurate at predicting aneurysm size and better at demonstrating thrombus, inflammatory aneurysms and any retroperitoneal bleeding or coexisting pathology. The relationship of the aneurysm to the renal arteries, coexisting renal artery stenosis and involvement of the iliac

arteries are easily demonstrated. Spiral CT is ideally suited for the postoperative evaluation of aortic stents, assessing both patency and any extravasation of contrast into the aneurysm sac.

Suggested technique for abdominal aorta

The technique is summarised in Box 6.5 and is discussed more fully below.

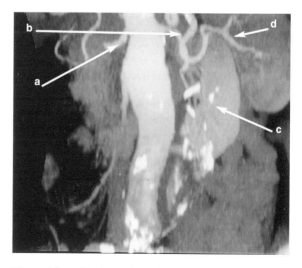

Figure 6.7 — Maximum intensity projection (MIP) of aorta aneurysm. a, right renal artery; b, left renal artery; c, left kidney d, splenic artery.

1. *Scanogram.*

2. *Precontrast scan.* This is low dose and low resolution and is performed to practise the prolonged breath-hold and to localise renal arteries and assess the required distance to be covered by the spiral. Commence the scan at the level of the diaphragm, with values 80 mA, 80 kV, 10 mm slice and pitch of 2

3. *Cardiac output estimate.* For the abdominal aorta a delay of 20–25 seconds is acceptable in the majority of patients. However if there is uncertainty about the patient's cardiac status, a test injection to assess cardiac output, indirectly or using the software provided on some scanners is recommended in order to customise the delay. For further details of the technique for cardiac output estimate, see the section on Renal artery stenosis (p. 92).

4. *Collimation.* For vessels running transversely a slice thickness of 3 mm or less is advisable, but for vessels running longitudinally a 5 mm slice is usually sufficient. So for the renal artery, a 3 mm slice with a pitch of 1 is suggested. Below the renal arteries a 5 mm slice with a pitch of 2 is used to cover the required distance. The patient should hold their breath while changing from one protocol to the other. No overlap of slices is needed. The patient can breathe out gently for the pelvis scan. Use 250–300 mA and 120–140 kV (depending on tube/scanner).

5. *Contrast.* The volume of contrast, which is injected at 2–4 ml/sec, should be sufficient to last the duration of the scan.

6. *Reconstruction.* Overlapping images should be obtained, reconstructing at least two images per rotation. The axial data is then manipulated to produce multiplanar and 3D images. The main techniques used are curved multiplanar reformats (MPR), surface shaded display (SSD), maximum intensity projections (MIP) and volume rendering (not available on all workstations). They all have advantages and limitations, and it is very important to refer to the original transaxial images if there are any questionable features on the 3D images. Curved MPRs take about 2–10 minutes, MIPs 10–40 minutes and SSDs 5–40 minutes depending on the amount of pre-editing performed.

Spleen

The spleen is shown well on CT. On unenhanced scans it has a CT number slightly less than that of the liver. The splenic vessels are seen well without contrast, but for optimal visualisation of the splenic parenchyma intravenous contrast should be administered, particularly if focal masses, such as lymphomatous deposits are suspected. If a slow injection of contrast is made, the spleen enhances uniformly. However, with bolus injections and early scanning, the spleen is non homogeneous (Figure 6.8) due to blood flow in different compartments. Care must be taken not to misinterpret this as focal abnormality and rescanning at 60 seconds will resolve the issue.

CT is the investigation of choice in splenic trauma and has advantages over ultrasound. When scanning for suspected splenic trauma, particularly using a spiral scanner the scans are performed 45–60 seconds after intravenous contrast to ensure that variable

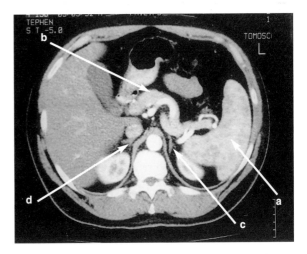

Figure 6.8 — Early scan through the spleen showing non-homogeneous enhancement (a) b, head of pancreas; (Note that the pancreas here is smooth in outline.) c, left adrenal; d, right adrenal.

parenchymal enhancement is not mistaken for a splenic laceration. In severe splenic trauma there is usually perisplenic fluid (Figure 6.9). The entire abdomen should be scanned to exclude significant liver, renal and mesenteric injury.

Adrenals

The technique is summarised in Box 6.6.

Anatomy

The adrenals lie within the perinephric fascia and are usually surrounded by an amount of fat sufficient to be readily visualised on CT. The right adrenal is usually seen on scans commencing 1–2 cm above the upper pole of the right kidney. It lies posterior to the inferior vena cava and between the crus of the diaphragm and the right lobe of the liver. The left adrenal lies at the same level or slightly more caudad, lying lateral to the aorta and the left crus and anteromedial to the upper pole of the left kidney. The adrenals extend 2–4 cm in

---

Box 6.6 — TECHNIQUE FOR ADRENALS
• Oral contrast
• Collimation 5 mm
• Field of view 250 mm
• Intravenous contrast not routinely required

---

a craniocaudad direction. The adrenals are seen as V shaped or as an inverted Y. The maximum width of the body measured perpendicular to the longitudinal axis is 0.8 mm on the left and 0.6 mm on the right and the thickness of the limbs should be less than 5 mm.

Adrenal masses

CT and, increasingly, magnetic resonance imaging (MRI) are the investigations of choice for adrenal pathology. CT will identify 100% of the adrenal glands if contiguous narrow collimation scans are used and adrenal masses are readily identified. Adrenal adenomas may be functioning or non functioning. A Conn's tumour is usually small, less than 2 cm and of low attenuation (0–10 HU). Other functioning adenomas are usually of higher attenuation, or the patients may have bilateral adrenal hyperplasia. Adrenal myelolipoma is a rare tumour which has characteristic features on CT as it contains fat (Figure 6.10) and no further investigation is required.

The major problem with adrenal imaging is the finding of an incidental adrenal mass. It is then important to know both the size and the attenuation of the mass. If the patient is biochemically normal, with no known malignancy, a lesion less than 3 cm is likely to be an adenoma. Even in the presence of known malignancy, if the mass is small with a CT number of less than 18 HU on an unenhanced scan it will be an adenoma. It is more of a problem if the patient has been given

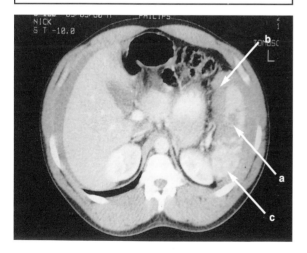

Figure 6.9 — Scan through upper abdomen of a patient with a splenic laceration (a). b, perisplenic haematoma; c, enhanced spleen.

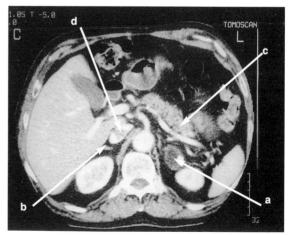

Figure 6.10 — Patient with myelolipoma containing fat (a). b, right adrenal; c, lobulated (compared with Figure 6.8) pancreas; d, Unopacified blood in the IVC, simulating thrombus in this early phase scan.

intravenous contrast, as the overlap between adenoma and non adenoma, i.e. metastasis, is wider on enhanced scans. Masses larger than 4 cm are malignant in 90% of cases. If there is doubt about the diagnosis, MRI may be helpful or CT-guided biopsy may be required.[18]

References

1. Brink JA .Technical aspects of helical (spiral) CT. *Radiol Clin North Am* 1995; **33**(5): 825–841.

2. Fishman EK Brooke J R *Spiral CT. Principles, techniques, and clinical applications*. New York, Raven Press.

3. Polacin A, Kalender WA, Marchal G. Evaluation of section sensitivity profiles and image noise in spiral CT. *Radiology* 1992; **185**: 29–35.

4. Fukuya T, Honda H, Hayashi T *et al*. Lymph node metastases: efficacy of detection with helical CT in patients with gastric cancer. *Radiology*. 1995; **197**: 705–711

5. Balthazar E, Freeny P, van Sonnenberg E. Imaging and intervention in acute pacreatitis. *Radiology* 1994; **193**: 297–306

6. Theoni RF, Blankenberg F. Pancreatic imaging. *Radiol Clin North Am*. 1993;. **31**(5): 1085–1113.

7. Hommeyer SC, Freeny PC, Crabo LG. Carcinoma of the head of the pancreas: evaluation of the pancreaticoduodenal veins with dynamic CT – potential for improved accuracy in staging. *Radiology*. 1995; **196**: 233–238

8. Zeman RK, Silverman PM, Ascher SM *et al*: Helical (spiral) CT of the pancreas and biliary tract. *Radiol Clin North Am* 1995; **33**(5): 887–902.

9. Rubin GD, Silverman SG. Helical (spiral) CT of the retroperitoneum. *Radiol Clin of North Am*. 1995; **33**(5): 903–932.

10. Szolar DH, KammerhuberF, Altzieble S *et al*. Multiphasic helical CT of the kidney: increased conspicuity for detection and characterisation of small (<3 cm) renal masses. *Radiology*. 1997; **202**: 211–217

11. Cochran ST, Krasny RM, Danovitch GM *et al*. Helical CT angiography for examination of living renal donors. *Am J Roentgenol*. 1997; **168**; 1569–1573

12. Galanski M, Prokop M, Chavan A, Schaefer CM, Jandelat K, Nischelsky JE. Renal arterial stenosis: helical CT angiography. *Radiology*.1993; **189**: 185–192.

13. Rubin GD, Dake MD, Napel S *et al*. Spiral CT of renal artery stenosis: comparison of three-dimensional rendering techniques. *Radiology* 1994; **190**: 181–189

14. Sommer FG, Brook JR, Rubin GD *et al*. Detection of ureteral calculi in patients with suspected renal colic: value of reformatted non contrast helical CT. *Am J Roentgenol* 1995; **165**: 509–513.

15. Smith RC, Rosenfield AT, Choe KA *et al*. Acute flank pain: comparison of non contrast enhanced CT and intravenous urography. *Radiology* 1995; **194**: 789–794.

16. Rubin GD, Dake MD, Semba CP. Current status of three-dimensional spiral CT scanning for imaging the vasculature. *Radiol Clin North Am*. 1995; **33**(1): 51–70.

17. Zeman RK, Silverman PM, Vieco PT, Costello P. CT angiography. *Am J Roentolog* 1995; **165**: 1079–1088.

18. Peppercorn PD, Reznek RH. State of the art CT and MRI of the adrenal gland. *Eur Radiol*.1997; **7**: 822–836.

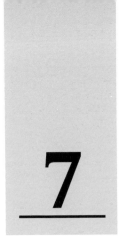

7

THE PELVIS

Emma Spouse and Suzanne Henwood

Introduction

Computed tomography (CT) and ultrasound (US) remain the predominant imaging modalities for the pelvis, although this could change as magnetic resonance imaging (MRI) sequences continue to improve. CT remains both cheaper and faster than MRI of the pelvis, whilst also providing better bony definition in most instances. Ultrasound, whilst cheaper than a CT examination of the pelvis, has yet to circumnavigate the problems of gas within the bowel and of imaging requiring the information provided by the use of contrast media.

Many patients will in fact undergo both an ultrasound and a CT examination of the pelvis. Ultrasound is the modality of first choice in many instances; it is fast, mobile, relatively cheap and does not employ ionising radiation. However, a CT examination will provide information unobtainable from an ultrasound scan. CT is not adversely affected by gas in the bowel, and has a larger field of view allowing clearer visualisation of structures and organs in relation to one another. In addition, obese patients, who are notoriously difficult to scan satisfactorily with ultrasound, can be visualised very nicely using CT (as long as they fit into the scanner). Surplus fat within the pelvis actually serves to delineate and isolate structures within the pelvis (and abdomen) from each other.

The advent of helical CT in recent years has revitalised dynamic contrast enhanced CT imaging, with rapid scanning times providing valuable diagnostic information in such areas as tumour definition and vascular delineation. Likewise, software programs continue to be developed, which improve the quality of three-dimensional (3D) reconstructions of the bony pelvis. Currently these programs require a workstation in addition to the CT scanner, as they are both time-consuming and disk space-hungry. However, it is possible to visualise such programs running concurrently, whilst continuing to image patients, in the not too distant future.

Inevitably the pelvis will often be examined in conjunction with the abdomen, as pathologies and conditions in one will often affect the other. For this reason, the text in this chapter specifies when certain pelvic pathologies demand CT scanning of both the abdomen and the pelvis. Techniques to demonstrate abdominal structures and pathologies, however, are discussed in detail in Chapter 6. Abdominal and pelvic scanning are also discussed comprehensively in Chiu *et al*.[1]

Patient preparation

Ideally the patient should have remained nil by mouth (NBM) for 2 hours prior to scanning if intravenous contrast is to be given and for 6 hours if oral contrast is required. Scanning can be carried out on unfasted patients if necessary.[2]

The pregnancy status of female patients under 50 years old should be checked. An alternative imaging procedure must be sought if there is any chance of pregnancy. The only exception is in cases of severe trauma.

As for all CT scanning, the area to be examined must be free from articles that may cause artefact on the resultant images. Ideally, the patient should be asked to undress and put on a cotton gown.

The patient must be given an adequate description of the scanning procedure in order that they may cooperate to the best of their ability.

If contrast agents are to be used, check that the patient has no contraindications to these before they are administered. Refer to the manufacturer's leaflet for a list of contraindications.

Oral contrast

Most pelvic scanning requires the use of oral contrast agents to demonstrate the bowel structures. The patient should be asked to arrive at least 1 hour before their scanning time, to drink 1 litre of oral contrast. If they drink over a shorter length of time, then the contrast will not have reached the large bowel by the time they are scanned, resulting in a more limited examination. Accelerators, such as 10 ml Maxalon, may be employed if necessary.

If the abdomen is to be included in the study, then one cupful of contrast should be saved to be drunk just before the patient is placed in the scanner (to demonstrate the stomach).

Note – Occasionally it may be necessary to introduce a little contrast medium rectally, particularly if the rectum, prostate, uterus or bladder are of particular interest.

CONTRAINDICATIONS

Some patients will be unable to tolerate oral contrast; the examination can still go ahead but, obviously, some information will be lost. Oral contrast can be administered via nasogastric tubes, medical conditions permitting; it is usually more convenient to take the oral contrast to the ward so that it can be administered by the nursing staff.

Care should be taken with patients suffering renal failure and on dialysis, as their fluid intake may be severely restricted. It is preferable to scan these patients just before their next dialysis session, and all administered fluids, (including intravenous (IV) contrast agents), must be carefully measured and documented.

Other contrast issues

Although the use of tampons for vaginal delineation in women and the use of gas for bladder enhancement has been documented,[1] along with the use of peritoneal soluble contrast[3] these methods are not routinely utilised. Abdominal and pelvic contrast enhancement is also discussed by Hamlin & Bergener[4] and in Chapter 2 of this book. Allen et al.[5] discuss some of the issues concerning the minimisation of contrast agent dose to optimal levels.

Patient position

The patient lies supine in the middle of the table (unless otherwise specified), with their arms above their head. A pillow or similar item can be used for supporting the head. Use pads and bands to support the arms. If the patient is unable to sustain this position for the duration of the scan, the arms may be folded high across the chest. The patient usually goes head first into the scanner.

If IV contrast is to be administered during the examination it is ideal to insert a Venflon and connect to the infusion pump before scanning begins. This helps prevent the likelihood of the patient moving position pre and post contrast administration and shortens the total scan time.

Contrast agents

Oral

Isopaque 100™ (100 mg/ml): 10 ml into 0.5 litres of water.

Intravenous

Omnipaque 350™: 60 – 80 mls diluted with 10 – 15 ml saline or sterile water solution.

A maximum of 110 ml of undiluted contrast can be given, e.g. for CT of aneurysms.

Although helical scanning, with its faster acquisition times, is said to reduce the quantities of IV contrast required, in reality this is not necessarily the case. Extra information can be gleaned using the so-called 'go and return' scan techniques, in the case of certain pathologies. In these instances more contrast agent might be delivered overall than would be given when scanning in one (usually superoinferior) direction. It is not unusual to deliver a total of 80 ml of contrast for one examination in this manner, i.e. 40 ml in each scan direction, rather than a mere 50 ml. When imaging structures such as the pancreas, 150 ml might be delivered, using a 'go, return and go' technique. See Chapter 6 for further information). Increased usage, and therefore the expense of contrast media can be minimised by diluting with normal saline solution. A typical dilution for an enhanced pelvic scan would be 60 ml Optiray 350™ mixed with 20 ml 0.9% normal saline solution.

Ideally IV contrast for pelvic CT scanning is administered via a pressure injector: 80 ml contrast-saline solution at a rate of 2 ml/sec with a 45-second delay; although these settings depend on the suspected pathology and/or diagnostic information required. This will vary between hospitals and with radiological preferences.

However, it is perfectly acceptable to hand inject the contrast agent if a pressure injector is unavailable. Ensure that both radiographer and radiologist know when the injection will be started and when the scanning will commence.

Refer to Chapter 2 for more detailed information on IV contrast media and their contraindications.

Safety

No one should remain in the scanning room during the scanning procedure unless it is absolutely necessary as in the case of injecting radiologist, or an accompanying nurse or relative if the patient is very sick and/or confused. All persons in the room during scanning, with the exception of the patient, must wear a lead rubber apron and stand as far away from the scanning aperture and gantry as possible. In this manner, the dose of unnecessary ionising radiation is minimised.

Check that all infusion lines, drips, catheter bags etc. will move with the patient during the scan and will not catch on anything as the table moves. Do not leave any-thing that might cause an artefact such as an infusion pump, either on or alongside the patient's pelvis. Make sure that the injection pump is as close to the patient as possible and that the connecting tube is long enough. The table will move a long way if the whole abdomen and pelvis is to be scanned.

The injecting radiologist should ensure that the Venflon in situ is patent, using saline, before the patient is connected to the pressure injector. Care must be taken to remove all air bubbles from the syringe con-taining contrast agent and from the connecting tube. Some pressure injectors have the facility to 'hand wind' the syringe plunger; this can be useful for drawing back until the operator sees venous blood in the connecting tube. The patient should be warned that they may well feel a hot flush and a metallic taste in the back of the throat as the contrast agent is injected.

Respiration issues

The patient requires clear instructions with regard to holding their breath. It is good practice to hyperventi-late the patient before commencing the scan. This can be done during the first 20 seconds of the injection. Hyperventilation often enables the patient to hold their breath for the duration of the whole scan, which can be up to 30 seconds during a spiral scan acquisi-tion, leading to better images. Patients unable to achieve this may start to breathe towards the end of the scan, usually whilst imaging the inferior pelvis. Respiration artefacts in this area are not as critical as in the abdomen.

Cluster acquisition of CT slice information is possible with spiral scanning software. Five or ten slices can be obtained per acquisition or breath hold. This technique provides a reasonable compromise. It is more achievable for the patient, in a situation where respiration artefact would severely affect the diag-nostic quality of the scans. This technique is also quicker than one slice acquisition per breath hold, making greater use of rapid contrast enhancement timing and techniques. However, differences in patient respiration between each cluster can cause some anatomy to be missed. This can be overcome by instructing the patient about the importance of similar respiration techniques beforehand, e.g. always holding their breath on inspiration of the same vol-ume of air.

Indeed, it is quite possible to obtain a reasonably diag-nostic pelvic scan in patients who are unable to suspend respiration at all. In these cases the patient should be told to keep their breathing as shallow as possible to keep respiration movement in the pelvis to a minimum. Another accepted technique, for imaging the whole abdomen and pelvis, is to suspend respiration whilst scanning the abdomen, with shallow breathing as the scan continues through the pelvis (assuming the scans are being obtained in a superoinferior, i.e. diaphragm to pubic symphysis, direction).

Many scanners will automatically ask the patient to hold their breath, using a prerecorded message. This needs to be synchronised to the injection of contrast and any delay programmed into the pressure injector. Other scanners will require that the operator asks the patient, via a microphone system, to hold their breath, although this is becoming less common.

Scan parameters

Normal scan parameters are shown in Table 7.1. These are general guidelines and will need to be adjusted according to the system in use and patient size and pathology.

If the pelvis is being scanned in conjunction with the abdomen, then the mAs setting can be increased from 200 to 250 at the level of the iliac crest and through the pelvis. In very large patients the kVp value may need to be increased to 130. This may prevent using a higher mAs value. Care must be taken not to overheat the X-ray tube, particularly in helical scanning as this will pro-duce cooling times, causing delays (usually at the most inopportune times!).

Conversely, when CT imaging the paediatric pelvis it is good technique to reduce the mAs value to 80. This reduces pelvic radiation dose substantially, without detectable differences in image quality.[6]

Table 7.1 – Normal scan parameters

kVp	90°–130
mAs	200–450
Table movement, mm (range)	10 (5–15)
Slice thickness, mm (range)	10 (5–15)
Field of view (FOV), cm	30–48
Matrix	512 × 256
Gantry tilt	0
Scan time, sec	5

The field of view (FOV) will vary according to the area under examination. For an average adult pelvis a 36 cm FOV is usually sufficient. If the patient is large this can be increased appropriately. To image the bladder, use FOV of about 30 cm.

Note – Image data will only be collected from the FOV selected. If the scan is obtained using the wrong FOV, e.g. 30 cm rather than 36 cm, the information outside the 30 cm FOV is lost and the scan will have to be repeated if information from the larger FOV is required. It is not possible to 'find' this information by manipulation of the raw data post scanning. Therefore, if in doubt as to the appropriate FOV, err on the large side. Too much information is better than too little and the images can be post processed to a smaller FOV using the raw data. However, an excessively large FOV should not be employed unnecessarily as this will reduce overall resolution.[7] Another alternative is to magnify the images retrospectively, although this will compromise image resolution of the hard copy.

Slice thickness and table movements will also vary according to requirements but 10/10 mm is the standard in pelvic imaging. In spiral scanning, the table will move continually throughout the scan and will move through the specified distance per slice thickness. The table will initially move to a position superior to the specified starting point in spiral scanning. The table will start to move, and gain continuous steady speed, before scanning commences at the selected cutline. Table movement can be selected and is usually of the order of 2–5 cm/sec. This will affect the other scan parameters.

Aspects of spiral scanning

Image resolution is not as good during spiral scanning as it is for the older, table movement 'scan, move, scan' techniques. This is because anatomical voxel detection and mapping cannot be as accurate during dynamic imaging compared to static scanning.[8] In static scanning, the CT table moves a specified distance and stops. The X-ray tubes then emit X-rays as they revolve around the patient, which in turn are detected as they emerge from the patient's mass. A computer system calculates the expected trajectory of a specific X-ray emission, and its actual emergent coordinates. The emergent secondary X-ray beam is thus located spatially, and given a grey scale value according to the calculated energy loss on its traverse through the patient. In the meantime, the table has moved again and the next scan has been undertaken.

In spiral scanning, this all becomes much more complicated. The table is moving continually; with the X-ray tubes emitting X-rays throughout the whole scan. The X-ray tubes rotate through 360 degrees and keep going by means of brushes that maintain continual contact, (rather than 360 degrees in one direction and then 360 degrees in the reverse direction as with older CT scanner technology), with the emergent beam X-ray detectors moving in synchronisation. This means that the patient (and their corresponding anatomical structures) have moved before the emergent X-rays from a particular voxel reach the detectors, making it much more difficult to calculate from where a particular secondary X-ray beam originates. In addition, this phenomenon also means that there is less information available from each individual voxel. The scanning computers use complicated algorithms to calculate these values.

However, there are several major advantages to using spiral scanning techniques in the pelvis:

- Scan times are generally quicker, which is beneficial to the patient and increases patient throughput on the machine.

- Respiration artefacts are kept to a minimum.

- It allows the use of 'go and return' scanning techniques. These are very useful in assessing tumour enhancement patterns after administration of a contrast agent, particularly in bladder pathologies and lymphadenopathy.

Direction of scan

The standard is to scan from an anatomically superior level to an inferior one. In the pelvis this means scanning from the level of the iliac crests through to the midpoint of the pubic symphysis. If the abdomen is to be included, it is usual to start at the level of the diaphragm. It is possible to vary slice thickness and table movement if scanning through the whole abdomen and pelvis. This technique will depend on patient pathology and the information required from the study. For example, for lymphoma follow-up, values of 15/15 mm through the abdomen and 10/10 mm through the pelvis may be used.

Care needs to be taken when spiral scanning, using a 'go and return' technique. The 'go' scan will usually follow the standard superior to inferior direction, and the 'return' scan the converse, i.e. inferior to superior. This needs to be remembered when imaging the scans onto hard copy for reporting. Different scanning centres inevitably develop their own imaging protocols, according to the preferences of individual radiologists.

There are exceptions to scanning in a superoinferior direction. For example, possible carcinoma of the bladder, post contrast, requires scanning in an inferosuperior direction. This technique should catch the first blush of contrast if a lesion is present. A spiral scanner could then be programmed to 'return' in the more usual superoinferior direction after a short delay.

Image artefacts

As with any other imaging modality, care must be taken to minimise the effects of artefacts on the resultant images. Common pelvic artefacts on CT include streaking effects from hip prostheses (Figure 7.1), streaking artefacts from oral contrast in the bowel and intravenous contrast reaching the bladder, and blurring artefacts from patient respiration and/or movement.

Respiration artefacts should be minimal in the pelvis. However, the abdomen and pelvis are often imaged together, with abdominal imaging requiring suspended respiration. If slice acquisition is single or cluster scanning, the unwell patient may find repeatedly holding their breath exhausting by the time their pelvis is being scanned. In spiral scanning, where the whole abdomen and pelvis can be imaged in one acquisition, the patient may be required to hold their breath for up to 30 seconds. This may be difficult for some people. To counteract potential problems it may be necessary to reduce

the imaging time further, or obtain the study in two acquisitions. Hyperventilating the patient immediately beforehand is also helpful.

A spiral scanning technique that may overcome this problem is to scan using 15/15 mm slice thickness and table movement (which will have a quicker scan time than the more usual 10/10 mm). Images can then be reconstructed, using the raw data post scanning, to 10/10 or even 5/5 mm slices. Remember that the raw data will be required to perform these reconstructions, as for all other data manipulation. It is not possible to reconstruct in this manner from archived images. A sensible precaution is to clear out the scanner's hard disk space before commencing the examination. Most scanners still require that the reconstructions be carried out fairly promptly to prevent the hard disk becoming unacceptably full for continuation of scanning. Imaging centres and radiology departments develop their own methods for dealing with raw data reconstruction, thereby avoiding raw data being removed before reconstructions have been undertaken.

Where a patient is unable to cooperate shallow respiration can be continued whilst scanning. Whilst this causes blurring artefacts in the abdomen, the pelvis may not be affected and a useful study obtained. (See also the section on Respiration issues, earlier in this chapter).

Artefacts may also be caused by catheters, intrauterine contraceptive devices (IUCDs) and biopsy needles. Whilst IUCDs can be clearly visible on CT scans (Figure 7.2), ultrasound should be used to identify the exact location of lost ones.

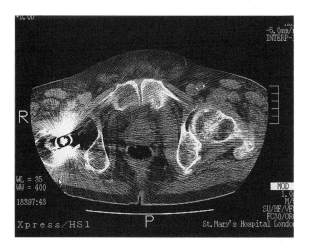

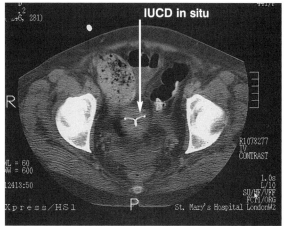

Figure 7.1 — Right hip prosthesis causing gross streaking artefacts.

Figure 7.2 — CT image showing intrauterine contraceptive device (IUCD).

Figure 7.3 shows a biopsy needle artefact. This scan was obtained during a CT-controlled biopsy of a mass, in the right iliac fossa, post pancreatic transplant.

Imaging

Most centres in the UK currently use laser imagers and 35 × 43 cm single-sided, laser-sensitive, emulsion film. Dry laser processors are superceding laser processors that use wet chemical solutions. The former take up less space, process as fast and largely eliminate the emission of harmful chemical fumes.

Generally, a format of 15 images per sheet is used for pelvic imaging. Conventionally, imaging starts at the anatomically superior slice, moving inferiorly. In the pelvis this means starting with the iliac crest and imaging down to the pubic symphysis. It is usual to include the anteroposterior (AP) planning scan, with cutlines, for ease of slice identification during reporting. If the use of contrast agents is not clear within the scan parameters on each image, it is important to annotate the scans appropriately, e.g. 'with oral and 60 ml IV contrast'.

The usual imaging parameters are window width (WW) 450–500 and window level (WL) 50, written as (450/50) (WW/WL).

These may require altering, as for instance this width and level might make the image look very grey and flat in a large patient. In this instance try 400/35, which are windowing parameters more usually employed for abdominal CT scans.

Techniques, images and pathologies in CT of the pelvis

All scans require an initial AP scanogram. Different scanners and manufacturers refer to initial scans differently; for instance as scanograms, scouts or topograms, but they are all the same thing – a scan from which the main scans are planned.

Figure 7.4 shows a scanogram with typical 10/10 mm slice thickness planning. Note the enormous inguinal hernia between this patient's legs. This highlights the need to check the scout scan carefully for useful information that may help to plan the main scans.

Anatomy of the pelvis

Figures 7.5–7.7 show normal male and female pelvic anatomy. A full review of normal male and female anatomy can be found in Chapter 11 of Chiu et al.[1]

Pelvic soft tissue pathologies

CARCINOMAS

CT will often be a means of staging, as well as diagnosing pelvic carcinomas. Lymph node involvement will be looked for and must therefore be included on the scans. Pelvic lymph nodes accompany the common iliac, external iliac and obturator vessels.[7] Lymph nodes are often difficult to visualise except when there is lymphadenopathy (which literally translates as lymph node involvement in a pathological process). Lymph nodes become

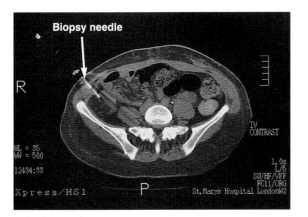

Figure 7.3 — Biposy needle artefact

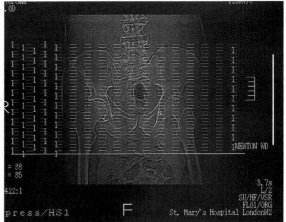

Figure 7.4 — Anterosuperior (AP) view of pelvis showing scanogram and cutlines.

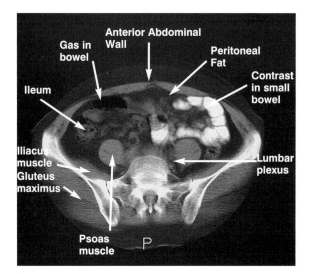

Figure 7.5 — Normal female anatomy at the level of the iliac crest.

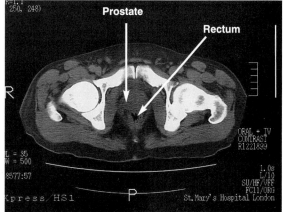

Figure 7.7 — Normal male anatomy at the level of the prostate.

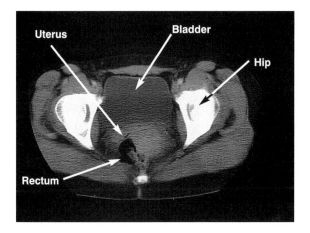

Figure 7.6 — Normal female anatomy at the level of the bladder and uterus.

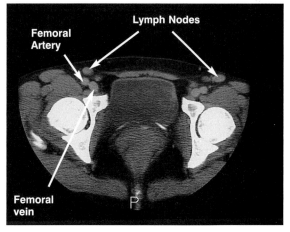

Figure 7.8 — CT image showing lymphadenopathy.

visible when they are enlarged, asymmetric or enhance after the administration of intravenous contrast.

Figure 7.8 indicates how difficult it can be to differentiate lymph nodes from femoral vessels, making IV contrast enhancement essential. Peak venous enhancement is generally between 3 and 7 minutes post injection.[9]

The proximity of pelvic structures and organs to each other makes good oral contrast imperative for adequate bowel demonstration; pelvic carcinomas usually invade neighbouring structures in the first instance.

MRI would now often be the imaging modality of choice, as this generally gives better soft tissue definition. However, MRI is expensive and there are contraindications, e.g. when patients have pacemakers, or magnetically susceptible implants or clips, or suffer from claustrophobia.

BLADDER

Figure 7.9 shows the bladder being displaced laterally by an anterior pelvic mass.

Figure 7.10 shows a urinary bag on the abdominal wall filling with contrast. The ilial conduit has also been visualised. This surgery was necessary following

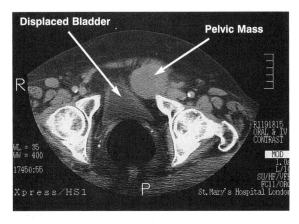

Figure 7.9 — Bladder displacement in a 65-year old woman.

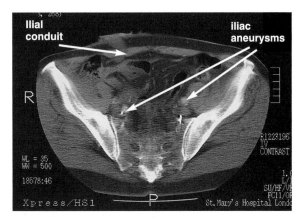

Figure 7.10 — Ilial conduit on anterior abdominal wall.

cystectomy, for bladder carcinoma, in this 69-year old man. The bilateral iliac aneurysms are an incidental finding. This highlights the fact that multiple disease processes and pathologies may be present and should, therefore, be looked for thoroughly before getting a patient off the scanning table, in case extra imaging is required.

The bladder is normally between 2 and 5 mm thick.[7] Figure 7.11 shows a transitional cell carcinoma with local invasion. CT is a good imaging modality to show local invasion but not for bladder carcinoma staging. This is because CT is unable to differentiate well between the bladder wall layers. MRI with gadolinium enhancement is more appropriate in this instance.

Adaptation of scanning technique for the bladder – Helical scanning is performed through area of interest, reconstructing 5/5 mm, with dynamic IV contrast. An optimal scan can be obtained using the 'go and return'

technique. If this is to be employed, start scanning at the pubic symphysis in an inferosuperior direction, at about 20 seconds after contrast delivery commences at a rate of 3 ml/second. Return immediately, in the superoinferior direction, to catch the second phase of contrast enhancement of the bladder.

CT images must include the whole bladder and rectum, i.e. scan to below the pubic symphysis. It is also essential to image the abdomen, to exclude invasion into the upper urinary tract.

Figue 7.12 shows a complicated postsurgical scan. There is an open, infected pelvic wound and multiple collateral vessels within the pelvis are also demonstrated.

CERVIX AND VAGINA

MRI is superior to CT visualisation of uterine and cervical carcinomas. The ovaries are rarely clearly delineated on CT.[10]

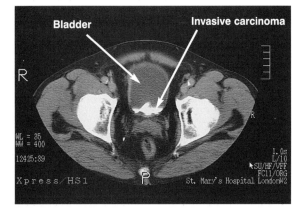

Figure 7.11 — Transitional cell carcinoma (TCC) of the bladder, with local invasion.

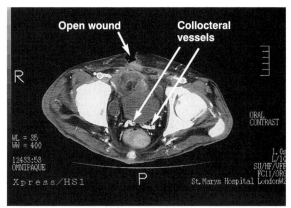

Figure 7.12 — Duodenal conduit to bladder.

Vaginal cancer with associated lymphadenopathy is shown in Figure 7.13. The huge lymph nodes indicate that this disease is well advanced.

Vaginal vault carcinoma is shown in Figure 7.14. The appearance of air within the vagina is abnormal and usually indicates intrapelvic malignancy.[11] In women with human immunodeficiency virus (HIV)-related carcinomas, the appearance of large, necrotic and rapidly growing lymph node metastases is now recognised as being diagnostic of acquired immunodeficiency syndrome (AIDS).[12] Other AIDS-related disorders manifested on CT are outlined by Kuhlman et al.[13]

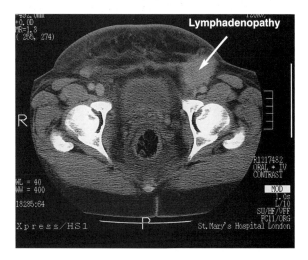

Figure 7.13 — Vaginal cancer with associated lymphadenopathy.

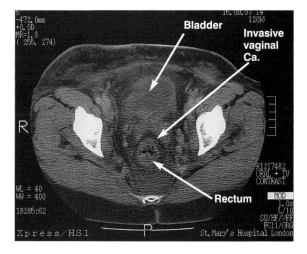

Figure 7.14 — Vaginal vault carcinoma.

PROSTATE

Figure 7.15 shows an enlarged prostate in a 74-year old man with urinary symptoms. If the prostate is seen more than 2 cm above the symphysis pubis, enlargement can be diagnosed. In men below 30 years of age, the craniocaudal diameter of the prostate is 3 cm; between 60 and 70 years it rises to 5 cm.[7] Latent prostate carcinomas, which are not the cause of death, are found in more than 70% of men over the age of 80 years; two-fifths of men over 65 years, who die from unrelated causes, are found to have prostatic cancer.[14]

TESTES

Ultrasound or MRI would be the examination of choice. However, CT is often carried out following surgery for teratomas (which are particularly aggressive) and seminomas. These disseminate further via the lymph system in the first instance and IV contrast can be used to enhance the lymph nodes.

Undescended testes - These patients are usually very young boys and ultrasound is the examination of choice. If the testes are not identified readily on ultrasound, MRI might prove illuminating.

The position of the seminal vesicles (Figure 7.16) is not fixed and can change slightly with patient position.

OVARIAN TUMOURS

The ovaries are normally only visible if they are enlarged. The most common primary malignant ovarian tumours are adenocarcinoma, serous or mucous cystadenocarcinoma and endometrioid carcinoma.[15]

Ascites is the most frequently observed pelvic fluid collection (Figure 7.17). It usually presents with a CT density value close to that of water on the Hounsfield scale (H), but can have a value of 10 to 30 H depending on its protein content.[7]

OVARIAN CYSTS

Ovarian cysts are diagnosed and analysed using ultrasound.

UTERUS

Figure 7.18 shows a relatively small uterine fibroid. The calcification within the uterine body is a common finding. Fibroids can be enormous, filling most of the pelvic cavity.

The bulky uterus in Figure 7.19 contains fluid, possibly from an endometrial carcinoma. The normal uterus often contains a central area of low attenuation.

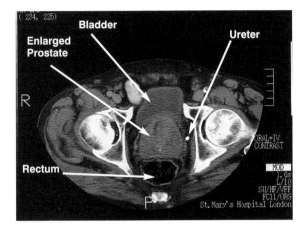

Figure 7.15 — Image showing prostatic enlargement.

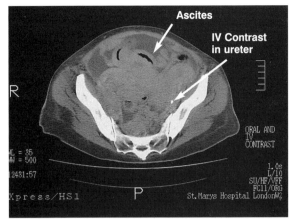

Figure 7.17 — Generalised ascites as a result of suspected ovarian malignancy.

RECTAL MASSES AND POLYPS

Note the obvious polypoid nature of the rectal mass in Figure 7.20.

VASCULAR PATHOLOGIES

Arteries have three layers to their walls. In aneurysms the arterial wall is weakened and these layers move apart, trapping blood between them. The scan of Figure 7.21 demonstrates well the false lumen of the aneurysm. The brightest part of the lumen is the aorta containing contrast media, whilst the darker enhancement shows slower blood flow in the false lumen. There are also peripheral calcifications in the wall of the vessel, another indicator of arterial disease.

For inguinal aneurysms see Figure 7.10. Iliac artery aneurysms are often mistaken for masses and it is therefore essential to use IV contrast during CT imaging.[16] There is often normal asymmetry in common iliac vein demonstration, due to differing obliquity of left and right,[17] which should not be confused with a mass.

HERNIA

Figure 7.22 shows an iliac hernia. In this patient, most of the small bowel has herniated through the inguinal and lower abdominal muscles. Hernias can cause the bowel to twist and become obstructed, creating further complications for the patient.

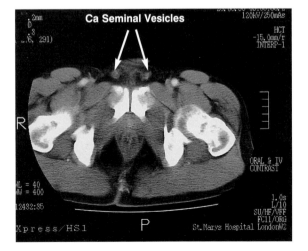

Figure 7.16 — Seminal vesicles.

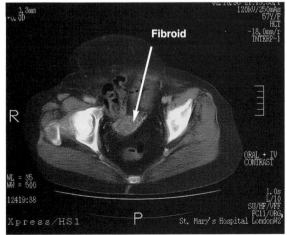

Figure 7.18 — Uterine fibroids

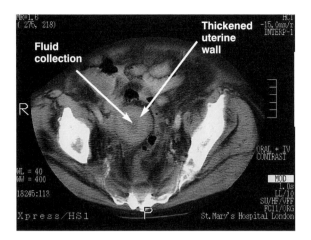

Figure 7.19 — Bulky uterus.

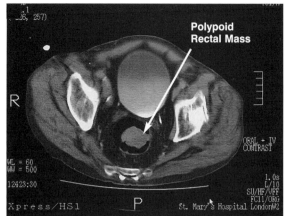

Figure 7.20 — Rectal mass.

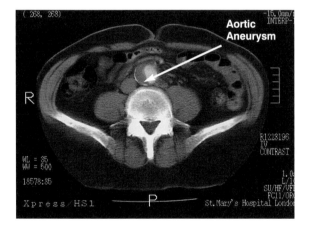

Figure 7.21 — Contrast-enhanced aortic aneurysm.

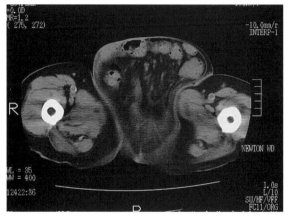

Figure 7.22 — Iliac hernia

FLUID COLLECTIONS AND ABSCESSES

Biopsy is necessary to confirm the diagnosis and to exclude possible malignancy. This may also alleviate the need for surgery. Abscesses and fluid collections can be drained under CT control quite easily, with an accuracy of over 90% and a very low complication rate.[18] Drains and fluid collection bags can be left in situ if necessary (Figure 7.23).

A fine needle biopsy, showing the needle trajectory, in which a 20 G true cut biopsy was undertaken, and is shown in Figure 7.24.

Note – The streaking artefact from the biopsy needle makes the needle look longer than it is in reality. This is a common artefact and needs to be taken into consid-

eration when using CT images to calculate measurements. (See the section on image artefacts earlier in this chapter).

See also Figure 7.17 for ascites and Figure 7.19 for uterine fluid collection.

Radiotherapy planning

CT is often used to plan a regime of radiotherapy treatment. This will only be undertaken by diagnostic radiographers in conjunction with therapeutic radiographers and physicists. At the planning stage the patient will have been diagnosed and will usually be well informed as to the problem for which they are to be treated. Radiotherapy planning is a vital stage for the patient's prognosis and must be undertaken with

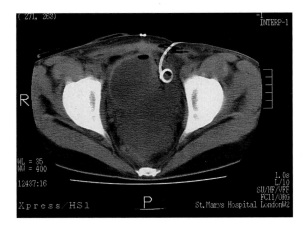

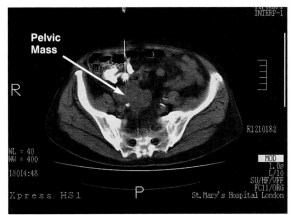

Figure 7.23 — Pigtail catheter draining pelvic fluid collection.

Figure 7.24 — Biopsy of pelvic mass.

great accuracy as well as diplomacy and good professional care.

High quality, accurate imaging is essential in ensuring that the diseased area to be treated can be targeted precisely, with minimal damage to surrounding healthy tissues.

PATIENT PREPARATION

The reader should refer again to the earlier section on patient preparation. The patient will need to wear a gown that is open to the relevant skin surface, e.g. open to the back for rectal tumours, open to the front for bladder tumours. The radiotherapists will usually have explained to the patient exactly what the imaging procedure entails.

The patient can breathe gently throughout scanning, as they will not be required to suspend respiration during radiotherapy treatment.

PATIENT POSITION

It is imperative that this resembles the treatment position, as far as is reasonably achievable. Often a special board is provided that fits into the curved scanning table top to produce a completely flat surface, or a flat table top can be purchased where significant numbers of planning CT scans are undertaken.

The patient lies as flat and as symmetrically as possible on the scanning table (either supine or prone). The patient is positioned accurately using two horizontal and one AP lasers and the patient's skin is then marked with indelible markers and radio-opaque markers (Figure 7.25).

If the patient is to undergo total body irradiation (TBI), e.g. for leukaemia, then they must be made as 'rectangular' as possible. This involves using sandbags and bandages, but this is the domain of the therapists and physicists. Radiation planning should always be undertaken with the guidance of these professionals.

Axial scans are taken of the pelvis (usually using 10/10 or 10/15), to check the markers are level. The carcinoma of the bladder is clearly demonstrated in Figure 7.26.

The bony pelvis

PATIENT PREPARATION

See the earlier section on Anatomy of the pelvis. The bony pelvis will often be imaged for trauma. For optimal scanning it is important to remove all items of clothing likely to cause artefact e.g. trousers or skirts with zips; these should be cut off the patient if necessary. Care must be taken to ensure that the patient lies as flat and as symmetrically as possible on the scanning table. Pain relief might be essential to enable this to be achieved in severe acute trauma.

SCANNING TECHNIQUE

Usually 10/10 mm will be sufficient. However, in trauma situations 5/5 mm may be required, through fracture sites e.g. acetabular fractures. Imaging must always include both soft tissue and bony windows.

For soft tissue windows: WL/WW is (450–500)/50.

For bony windows: WL/WW is (3000–4000)/60.

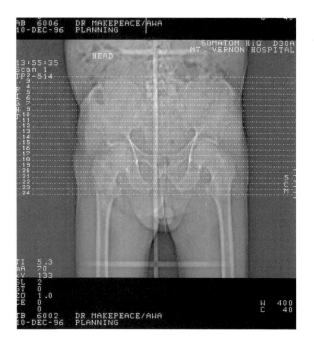

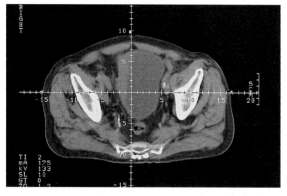

Figure 7.26 — Axial section through tumour demonstrating radio-opaque markers in situ.

acetabulum and left femoral head as a consequence of an old traumatic fracture.

Figure 7.28 shows a pelvic fracture of the pubic ramus. This clearly demonstrates an acute break in the bony cortex, along with pelvic asymmetry. Consistent with normal pelvic trauma expectations, this patient also had other pelvic fractures including the alar wing and sacrum, i.e. multiple breaks in the pelvic ring, as discussed by Pitt *et al*[19] and Buckley & Burkus.[20] Other areas of disruption are shown in images from the same patient (Figures 7.29 and 7.30). The left sacroiliac joint is noticeably wider than that on the right.

It is important to note that in CT imaging of the traumatically injured pelvis, soft tissue windows are always required to eliminate bladder and ureteric involvement. CT is also useful in determining the presence or

Figure 7.25 — AP scanogram demonstrating three radio-opaque markers in situ on the skin surface.

AVASCULAR NECROSIS

Both hips should be scanned for direct comparison. MRI is the imaging modality of choice as CT is not as sensitive to subtle necrotic changes within the femoral head.

FRACTURES

A pelvic fracture is demonstrated in Figure 7.27. This 74-year old man had a deformed symphysis,

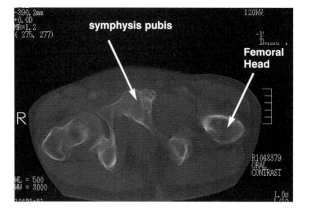

Figure 7.27 — Bony windows demonstrating an old pelvic fracture.

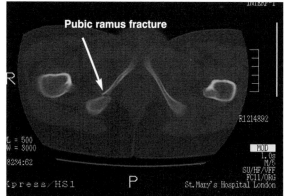

Figure 7.28 — Pelvic fracture of the pubic ramus.

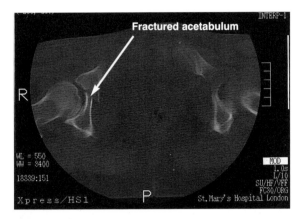

Figure 7.29 — Acetabular fracture.

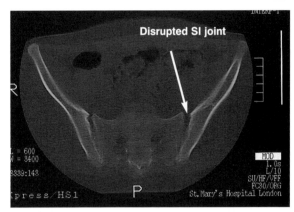

Figure 7.30 — Disrupted sacroiliac joint.

absence of bleeding.[21] A rapid infusion of contrast agent improves the visualisation of haematoma,[22] which should be suspected in patients presenting with iliac vein obstruction after blunt pelvic trauma, even in the absence of fractures.[23]

Some departments have the computer hardware and software available to manipulate the raw data and produce three-dimensional representations of the anatomy scanned. This can be extremely useful in the case of complex pelvic fractures where surgical intervention is necessary, as well as in the paediatric patient.[24]

PELVIMETRY

Pelvimetric measurements of the pelvis can be taken from CT images. Ideally, the patient should be scanned post partum, i.e. before an ensuing pregnancy, to avoid irradiation of the foetus. CT has been found to deliver less radiation to the foetus than conventional plain film pelvimetry.[25,26] However, MR would now be the examination of choice, unless expedience and expense dictate otherwise.[27] In reality, it would be somewhat exceptional to undertake a pelvimetric examination, using ionising radiation, on a pregnant woman in the late 1990s. Recent thinking has also suggested that there is little benefit in undertaking prophylactic pelvimetry, as statistically there is little change in birth outcomes: i.e. the caesarean rate does not change significantly, whether or not a woman has had problems resulting from cephalopelvic disproportion in a previous labour.[28]

The patient is prepared as for the usual CT of pelvis. Ideally they should lie prone. However, if she is heavily pregnant this option would not be feasible. Care must be taken to ensure that the patient lies exactly straight on the scanning table, in order that accurate measurements can be taken from the images.

A lateral scanogram only is performed (Figure 7.31). Use a conventional pelvic scanogram protocol and change from AP to lateral parameters. Employ the minimum imaging parameters possible to obtain a good diagnostic image, to keep the ionising radiation dose as low as reasonably achievable.

Measurements are taken from the anterior tip of the first sacral vertebra to the superior posterior point of the pubic symphysis (1), the pelvic inlet, and from the anterior tip of the last fixed sacral segment to the inferior posterior point of the pubic symphysis (2), the pelvic outlet (Figure 7.32). The lengths and angles of these lines indicate whether or not the baby (dependent on size, of course) can be delivered via the birth canal.

ACKNOWLEDGEMENTS

The authors are grateful to Pat Fernie, Superintendent Radiographer, Paul Strickland Scanner Centre, for the radiotherapy planning images, and to the radiographers operating the CT scanner at St Mary's Hospital, Paddington, London, between 1995 and 1997 for all other images.

References

1. Chui LC, Lipacamon JD & Yiu-Chiu VS. *Clinical computed tomography for the technologist* (2nd edn). New York, Raven Press 1995, chs 10,11.

2. Gedroyc W, Rankin S. *Practical CT techniques*. London: Springer-Verlag, 1992

3. Frasci G, Contino A, Iaffaioli RV, Mastrantonio P, Conforti S,. Persico G. Computerized tomography of the abdmoen and pelvis with peritoneal administration of soluble contrast (IPC-CT) in detection of residual disease for patients with ovarian cancer. *Gynecol Oncol.* 1994; **52**(2): 154–160.

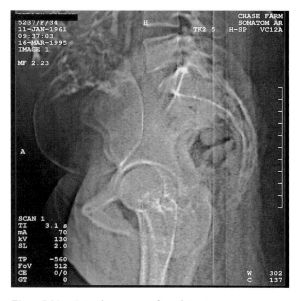

Figure 7.31 — Lateral scanogram for pelvimetry.

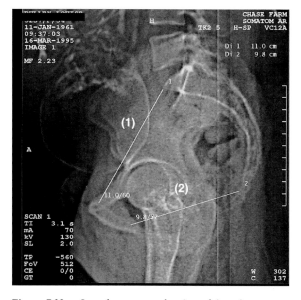

Figure 7.32 — Lateral scanogram showing pelvimetric measurements.

4. Hamlin DJ. Burgener FA. Positive and negative contrast agents in CT evaluation of the abdomen and pelvis. *Computed Tomogr.*1981; **5**: 82–90, 1981

5. Allen DA., Stoupis C., Torres GM., Call GA, Litwiller TL,. Ros PR. Dose optimization of nonionic contrast agent in dynamic computed tomography scanning of the abdomen and pelvis. *Clin Imaging.* 1994; **18**(1): 72–74.

6. Kamel IR, Hernandez RJ, Martin JE, Schlesinger AE, Niklason L, Guire KE. Radiation dose reduction in CT of the pediatric pelvis. *Radiology.* 1994; **190**: 683–687.

7. Moss AA, Gamsu G, Genant HK *Computed tomography of the body with magnetic resonance imaging. Abdomen and pelvis.(2nd edn).* Philadelphia: WB Saunders, 1992, vol 3.

8. Seeram E. Computed tomography - *Physical principles, clinical applications and quality control.* Philadelphia: WB Saunders, 1994.

9. Teefey SA, Baron RL, Schulte SJ, Shuman WP Differentiating pelvic veins and enlarged lymph nodes: optimal CT techniques. *Radiology.* 1990; **175**(3): 683–685.

10. Kim SH, Choi BI, Lee HP, Kang SB, Choi YM, Han MC, Kim CW Uterine cervical carcinoma: comparison of CT and MR findings. *Radiology.* 1990; **175**(1): 45–51.

11. Hadar H, Kornreich L, Heifetz M, Herskovitz P, Horev G. Air in vagina. Indicator of intrapelvic pathology on CT [Abstract]. *Acta Radiol.*1991; **32**(3): 170–173.

12. McDermott VG, Langer JE, Schiebler ML. Case report: HIV-related rapidly progressive carcinoma of the cervix. *Clin Radio.*1994; **49**(12): 896–898.

13. Kuhlman JE, Browne D Shermak M, Hamper UM, Zerhouni EA, Fishman EK. Retroperitoneal and pelvic CT of patients with AIDS: primary and secondary involvement of the genitourinary tract. *Radiographics.* 1991; **11**(3): 473–483.

14. Siddall R. Time to screen for prostate cancer? *New Scientist.* 1993 27–30

15. Brammer HM., Buck JL, Hayes W, Sheth S, Tavassoli FA. Maligant germ cell tumors of the ovary; radiologic – pathologic correlation. *Radiographics.* 1990; **10**: 715–724.

16. Arenson AM, Graham R, Hamilton P, Mitchell S. Iliac artery aneurysms presenting as large pelvic masses. *Australas Radiol.* 1989; **33** (3): 229–232.

17. Meanock CI, Ward CS, Williams MP. A potential pitfall of pelvic computed tomography. *Br J Radio.* 1988; **61**(727): 584–585.

18. Murphy FB, Bernadino ME, Interventional computed tomography [Review] *Curr Problems Diagn Radiol* 1988; **17**(4): 121–154.

19. Pitt MJ, Ruth JT, Benjamin JB. Trauma to the pelvic ring and acetabulum. *Semin Roentgenol.* 1992; **27**(4): 299–318.

20. Buckley SL,. Burkus JK. Computerized axial tomography of pelvic ring fractures. *J Trauma.* 1987; **27**(5): 496–502.

21. Cerva DS, Mirvis SE, Shanmuganathan K, Kelly IM, Pais SO. Detection of bleeding in patients with major pelvic fractures: value of contrast enhanced CT. *Am J Roentgenol.* 1996; **166**(1): 131–135.

22. Roberts JL, Dalen K, Bosanko CM, Jafir SZ. CT in abdominal and pelvic trauma. *Radiographics.* 1993; **13**(4): 735–752.

23. Baumgartner FJ, Goodnight J, Nordestgaard AG, White G. High grade occlusion of the iliac vein by a traumatic pelvic hematoma without fracture [Abstract]. *Klin Wochenschr.* 1990; **68**(12): 619–622.

24. Magid D, Fishman EK, Ney DR, Kuhlman JE, Frantz KM, Sponseller PD. Acetabular and pelvic fractures in the pediatric patient: value of two- and three-dimensional imaging. *J Pediat Orthoped.* 1992; **12**(5): 621–625.

25. Raman S, Samuel D, Suresh K. A comparative study of x-ray pelvimetry and CT pelvimetry. *Austr NZ J Obstet Gynaeco* 1991; **31**(3): 217–220.

26. Shrimpton PC, Jones DG, Hillier MC, Wall BF, Le Heron JC, Faulkner K. Survey of CT practice in the UK. National Radiological Protection Board/HMSO, 1991. Part 2: dosimetric aspects.

27. O'Reilly MAR, Bate JR. The use of MRI in obstetric pelvimetry. *Rad Magazine* 1997; **23**(269): 34.

28. American Federation of Family Practitioners (AFFP) *Prevention, recognition and management of dystocia. ALSO (advanced life support in obstetrics and gynaecology) course manual.* 1997

Index